FERTILITY DIET COOKBOOK FOR WOMEN

The Best Recipes to Reduce Inflammation, Balance Hormones and Boost Conception

Olivia Smith

Copyright © 2023 Olivia Smith

All rights reserved. No part of this book may be reproduced, stored, or transmitted in any form or by any means, electronic, mechanical, photocopying, recording, scanning, or otherwise, without the prior written permission of the copyright owner.

This book contains information that is protected by intellectual property laws and is the sole property of the author. Any unauthorized reprint or use of this material is prohibited.

This book is a work of non-fiction and the views expressed herein are the sole responsibility of the author. Any product, company, or organization mentioned herein is the trademark of their respective owners.

This book is provided "as is" without any express or implied warranties. While every effort has been made to ensure the accuracy of the information contained herein, the author assumes no responsibility for errors or omissions.

Published in the United States of America.

TABLE OF CONTENT

INTRODUCTION 7

PART 1: 11
    Understanding the Fertility Diet 11

CHAPTER 1 13
    What is Fertility Diet? 13
    How Diet Can Improve Fertility? 13

CHAPTER 2 16
    Eating a Fertility Diet 17
    Benefits of Eating a Fertility Diet 18

CHAPTER 3 21
    Foods to Avoid in Order to Conceive 21
    Foods to Eat in Order to Conceive 23

PART 2: 25
    Recipes to Reduce Inflammation and Balance Hormones 25

CHAPTER 4 26
    Anti-inflammation Meal Plan 26
    Day 1: 26
    Day 2: 29
    Day 3: 31
    Day 4: 34
    Day 5: 37
    Day 6: 39
    Day 7: 42

CHAPTER 5 45
    Hormone Balancing Diet Meal Plan 45
    Day 1 45

Day 2 49

Day 3 52

Day 4 55

Day 5 58

Day 6 62

Day 7 65

Part 3: 69

Boosting Fertility with Supplements and Herbs 69

CHAPTER 6 70

Supplements to Boost Fertility 70

CHAPTER 7 73

Herbal Remedies for Infertility 73

CHAPTER 8 75

FERTILITY RECIPES 75

BREAKFAST 75

   1. Omelet with Avocado, Tomato, and Cheese: 75

   2. French Toast with Nut Butter and Berries: 76

   3. Scrambled Eggs with Spinach and Feta: 77

   4. Yogurt Bowl with Granola and Honey: 77

   5. Breakfast Smoothie Bowl: 78

   6. Overnight Oats with Berries: 79

   7. Breakfast Burrito with Eggs and Black Beans: 79

   8. Apple-Cinnamon Oatmeal: 80

   9. Breakfast Quesadilla with Eggs and Peppers: 81

   10. Egg Muffins with Spinach and Cheese: 82

LUNCH 83

   1. Mediterranean Quinoa Bowl - Prep time: 15 minutes 83

   2. Thai Peanut Noodle Bowl - Prep time: 15 minutes 84

3. Egg and Avocado Toast: Prep time: 10 minutes 84

4. Lemon Garlic Shrimp: Prep time: 10 minutes 85

5. Greek Salad Bowl - Prep time: 10 minutes 86

6. Grilled Vegetable Wrap: Prep time: 15 minutes 87

7. Baked Sweet Potato - Prep time: 10 minutes 87

8. Avocado Toast with Fried Egg - Prep time: 10 minutes 88

9. Chickpea Salad - Prep time: 10 minutes 89

10. Roasted Vegetable Bowl - Prep time: 20 minutes 89

DINNER 91

1. Pesto Chicken, Tomato, and Asparagus Skewers – Prep Time: 15 minutes 91

2. Feta and Spinach Stuffed Mushrooms – Prep Time: 15 minutes 92

3. Baked Salmon with Herbed Yogurt Sauce – Prep Time: 10 minutes .. 92

4. Eggplant Parmesan – Prep Time: 15 minutes 93

5. Baked Cod with Lemon and Parsley – Prep Time: 15 minutes 94

6. Roasted Sweet Potato Salad – Prep Time: 20 minutes...................... 95

7. Zucchini Noodles with Tomato Alfredo Sauce – Prep Time: 10 minutes 96

8. Garlic Butter Shrimp – Prep Time: 10 minutes 97

9. Baked Zucchini Fritters – Prep Time: 15 minutes 97

10. Baked Tofu with Sweet and Spicy Glaze – Prep Time: 10 minutes ... 98

SNACK 100

1. Avocado and Egg Toast: 100

2. Apple and Cheese Skewers: 100

3. Greek Yogurt and Fruit Parfait: 101

4. Trail Mix: 102

5. Hummus and Veggies: 102

6. Peanut Butter and Banana Toast: 103

    7. Quinoa and Veggies: 104

    8. Dark Chocolate and Almond Butter Bites: 104

    9. Smoothie: 105

    10. Avocado Toast with Egg: 106

DESSERTS 107

    1. Carrot Cake Cupcakes with Cream Cheese Frosting: 107

    2. Chocolate Chip Cookie Cake: 108

    3. Apple Pie Bars: 109

    4. Blueberry Cheesecake Bars: 110

    5. Strawberry Shortcake Trifle: 111

    6. Banana Pudding Parfaits: 112

    7. Lemon Bars: 113

    8. Raspberry Truffles: 114

    9. Chocolate Mousse Cake: 114

    10. Coconut Cream Pie: 115

SMOOTHIES 117

    1. Berry Pomegranate Smoothie 117

    2. Spinach Mango Smoothie 117

    3. Avocado Banana Smoothie 117

    4. Chocolate Oats Smoothie 118

    5. Orange Carrot Smoothie 118

    6. Peach Coconut Smoothie 119

    7. Green Tea Smoothie 119

    8. Pineapple Coconut Smoothie 119

    9. Apple Cinnamon Smoothie 120

    10. Banana Oat Smoothie 120

CONCLUSION 121

INTRODUCTION

Laureen Fertility Story:

Laureen was a married woman in her mid-thirties, who had been trying to conceive for more than 10 years. She had tried all the conventional treatments, but nothing had worked for her.

Desperate for a solution, she decided to try something new and came across my fertility diet recipes. She began following my advice and recipes for a balanced diet, full of foods that would promote fertility and help her conceive.

At first, Laureen found following the diet difficult. She was used to eating processed food and junk food, and had never paid much attention to her diet before. But she was determined to make this work, and so she persevered.

Laureen found that by following my diet plan, she felt healthier, more energized, and had more mental clarity. She also found that she was losing weight, which was a nice side effect.

After a few months, Laureen noticed that her menstrual cycle was becoming more regular. She was also feeling more fertile, and it seemed that all the changes she had made to her diet were having an effect.

Finally, after 10 years of trying, Laureen found that she was pregnant! She was overjoyed and couldn't believe that it had actually worked.

It was clear that the fertility diet recipes I had given her had made the difference. By eating foods that promote fertility, Laureen was able to conceive easily and overcome 10 years of barrenness.

She was so grateful to me and shared her story with her friends and family. She told them that if they were having trouble conceiving, then they should definitely try following my fertility diet recipes.

Laureen was proof that it worked, and that it could be the answer to many couples' fertility struggles. With determination and a balanced diet full of fertility-promoting foods, Laureen was able to conceive easily and overcome 10 years of barrenness.

BEVERLY Fertility story:

Beverly Grayer had been struggling to conceive for three years. She had a history of hormonal imbalances, and she had seen countless doctors and specialists in her attempt to get pregnant. Nothing seemed to work, and she was beginning to lose hope.

One day, she heard about my Fertility Diet Recipes and decided to give it a try. She was skeptical at first, but she figured she had nothing to lose.

She began following the recipes and was amazed at how quickly her body began to adjust. Within a matter of weeks, she could feel the difference in her energy levels and her overall health. She was also having fewer issues with hormone imbalances.

Beverly was amazed at the results she was getting, and after a few months, she was able to conceive. She was so relieved and grateful to finally be pregnant.

She continued to follow the recipes throughout her pregnancy and was able to maintain her healthy lifestyle. She was still having fewer issues with hormonal imbalances and her pregnancy proceeded without any complications.

After the birth of her child, Beverly was back on the diet and felt better than ever. She was so happy to have overcome her fertility issues and to be a mother.

She continued to follow the recipes for the next few years, and her family was able to enjoy the benefits of her healthy lifestyle. Beverly was so grateful for the knowledge she had gained through my Fertility Diet Recipes, and she was ecstatic that she had been able to overcome her three years of hormonal imbalances.

Her story is a testament to the power of following a healthy diet and lifestyle. She is proof that it is possible to overcome fertility issues and finally become a mother.

This book is designed to help you understand the power of nutrition and how it can help you conceive and have a healthy pregnancy.

We have compiled delicious, easy-to-follow recipes that are designed to reduce inflammation, balance hormones, and increase fertility. Each recipe is packed with nutrient-dense ingredients that provide the essential vitamins, minerals, and antioxidants that will support your reproductive health and help you conceive.

We understand that it can be difficult to make changes to your diet and lifestyle when you are trying to conceive. That's why we have made sure to include recipes that are not only nutritious, but also easy to prepare and delicious. We want to make sure that you enjoy the journey to conception and can do so without sacrificing flavor.

We hope that this book will provide you with the tools and knowledge to start nourishing your body and optimizing your fertility so that you can have a healthy pregnancy and bring a beautiful baby into the world.

PART 1:

Understanding the Fertility Diet

The Fertility Diet is an eating plan created by researchers at the Harvard School of Public Health. It is based on findings from the Nurses' Health Study, a long-term study of diet and health outcomes of over 100,000 female nurses. The diet emphasizes fruits, vegetables, whole grains, beans, and other plant-based foods. It also recommends limiting unhealthy fats and refined carbohydrates, as well as avoiding processed and packaged foods.

The goal of the Fertility Diet is to improve fertility and reduce the risk of ovulatory infertility. Research in the Nurses' Health Study found that women who followed the diet had an improved chance of becoming pregnant, and a decreased risk of ovulatory infertility.

The diet has several components, including:

Eating more fruits and vegetables: The diet recommends eating five or more servings of fruits and vegetables each day.

Eating whole grains: Eating at least three servings of whole grains, such as oats and brown rice, is also recommended.

Limiting unhealthy fats: The diet recommends limiting unhealthy fats, such as trans fats, saturated fats, and hydrogenated oils.

Limiting refined carbohydrates: The diet recommends limiting refined carbohydrates, such as white bread, white rice, and white pasta.

Eating more fiber: The diet recommends eating high-fiber foods, such as beans, lentils, and nuts.

Eating more plant-based protein: The diet recommends eating plant-based proteins, such as beans, lentils, nuts, and seeds.

Limiting processed and packaged foods: The diet recommends avoiding processed and packaged foods, such as frozen meals, fast food, and canned goods.

In addition to the diet, the Fertility Diet recommends regular physical activity and stress reduction to improve fertility.

Overall, the Fertility Diet is a healthy, balanced eating plan that emphasizes a variety of fruits, vegetables, and whole grains. It is a safe and effective way to improve fertility and reduce the risk of ovulatory infertility.

CHAPTER 1

What is Fertility Diet?

A fertility diet is a type of diet specifically designed to help women boost their fertility and increase the chances of conception. This diet consists of specific foods that are thought to support reproductive health in women.

Eating a fertility diet can help nourish the body and provide essential nutrients for optimal fertility, including vitamins, minerals, antioxidants, healthy fats, and proteins. The fertility diet is also believed to reduce inflammation and oxidative stress, which can interfere with a woman's ability to conceive.

How Diet Can Improve Fertility?

When it comes to improving fertility and increasing the chances of conceiving, diet plays an important role. Many couples who are trying to conceive may not realize how much their eating habits can actually influence their fertility and reproductive health. With the right dietary changes, couples can significantly increase their chances of conceiving.

Fertility experts suggest that couples who are trying to conceive should focus on eating more nutrient-rich and balanced meals. This means eating an array of healthy and whole foods including fruits, vegetables, lean proteins, whole grains, and healthy fats.

Eating a variety of foods will help to ensure that you are getting all the essential vitamins and minerals that your body needs to support a healthy reproductive system.

Research suggests that eating a diet rich in antioxidants can help to improve fertility. Antioxidants can help to reduce oxidative stress in the body, which can have a negative impact on fertility. Eating antioxidant-rich foods such as fruits, vegetables, nuts, and seeds can help to reduce oxidative stress and improve fertility.

Eating a diet that is rich in omega-3 fatty acids can also help to improve fertility. Omega-3 fatty acids are important for reproductive health and are found in foods such as fish, flaxseeds, and chia seeds. Eating more of these foods can help to improve fertility by promoting healthy ovulation and improving egg quality.

It is also important to ensure that you are eating enough calories and not under eating. Eating too few calories can lead to hormonal imbalances, which can interfere with fertility. To ensure that you are getting enough calories, focus on eating nutrient-dense foods such as nuts, seeds, legumes, and whole grains.

In addition to eating a balanced and nutrient-rich diet, it is important to reduce the amount of processed foods that you eat. Processed foods are often high in unhealthy fats and added sugars, which can have a negative impact on fertility. Instead, focus on eating more whole foods and less processed foods.

Finally, it is important to stay hydrated. Drinking plenty of water can help to support fertility by helping to regulate hormones and improving blood flow to the reproductive organs. Staying hydrated can also help to reduce stress, which can have a positive impact on fertility.

Making simple dietary changes can make a big difference when it comes to improving fertility. Eating a nutrient-rich diet can help to promote a healthy reproductive system and increase the chances of conceiving. Couples who are trying to conceive should focus on eating a balanced and varied diet, eating plenty of antioxidants, and reducing processed foods. Staying hydrated is also important for supporting fertility. By making small dietary changes, couples can increase their chances of conceiving and having a healthy pregnancy.

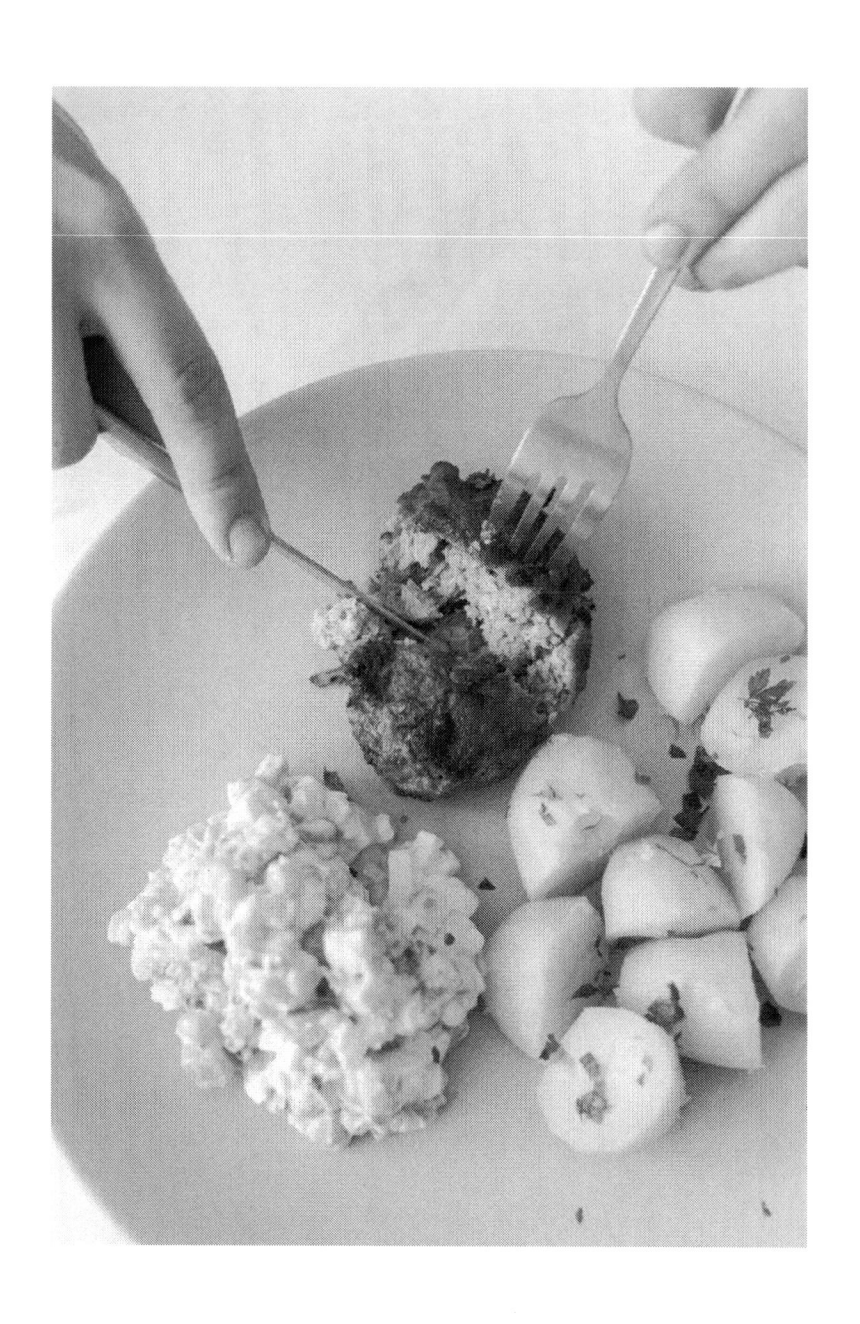

CHAPTER 2

Eating a Fertility Diet

Eating a Fertility Diet is an important step that many women are taking to increase their chances of conceiving and having a healthy pregnancy. A fertility diet is simply a well-balanced diet that includes foods that are known to promote reproductive health. This type of diet has been used for centuries to boost fertility and improve the chances of having a healthy baby.

The first step to eating a fertility diet is to make sure you are getting enough of the essential vitamins and minerals that are needed to support a healthy reproductive system. This includes vitamins A, C, D, E, K, folate, calcium, zinc, and selenium. All of these are necessary for healthy egg development and ovulation, as well as for a healthy sperm count and motility. Eating foods that are rich in these vitamins and minerals can help to ensure that your body has what it needs to support a healthy pregnancy.

Another important part of eating a fertility diet is to get enough protein. Protein provides the building blocks for healthy eggs and sperm, and is essential for a healthy reproductive system. Eating a variety of lean proteins, such as fish, poultry, and legumes, can help to ensure that your body has all the necessary nutrients for healthy fertility.

In addition to getting enough of the essential vitamins and minerals, eating a fertility diet also involves incorporating certain foods that are known to support a healthy reproductive system. These include foods that are high in antioxidants, such as berries, dark leafy greens, and nuts. Antioxidants help to protect the body from free radical damage, which can interfere with fertility. Other foods that are beneficial for fertility include foods high in omega-3 fatty acids, such as fatty fish, flaxseeds, and walnuts.

Finally, eating a fertility diet also means avoiding certain foods that can interfere with fertility. These include foods that processed, refined sugars, and trans fats. These types of foods can interfere with hormone balance and can reduce the chances of conception. It is best to avoid these types of foods as much as possible when trying to conceive.

Eating a fertility diet is a great way to make sure that your body is getting all the nutrients it needs to promote a healthy reproductive system. Eating the right foods and avoiding certain foods that can interfere with fertility can help to increase the chances of having a healthy pregnancy. Making sure that you are getting enough of the essential vitamins and minerals, as well as incorporating foods that are known to support a healthy reproductive system, can make all the changes when it comes to your fertility.

Benefits of Eating a Fertility Diet

Eating a fertility diet is essential for any woman who is trying to conceive. A fertility diet is a way of eating that helps to create a healthy and balanced environment in the body to support conception and a healthy pregnancy. Eating a fertility diet can provide many benefits for women, ranging from improved overall health and fertility to increased chances of conceiving.

One of the main benefits of eating a fertility diet is improved overall health. Eating a fertility diet can help to improve overall health by providing the body with the essential vitamins, minerals and nutrients needed to support a healthy reproductive system. Eating a fertility diet can also help to maintain a healthy weight, which is important for overall health and fertility. Eating a fertility diet can also help to reduce the risk of certain diseases and conditions, such as diabetes and heart disease.

Eating a fertility diet can also help to improve fertility. Eating a fertility diet can help to create a healthy hormonal balance in the body, which is essential for fertility. Eating a fertility diet can also help to reduce inflammation in the body, which can interfere with the ability to conceive. Eating a fertility diet can also help to increase the production of healthy sperm and eggs, which are both essential for conception.

Eating a fertility diet can also increase the chances of conceiving. Eating a fertility diet can help to provide the body with the essential nutrients needed to support conception and a healthy pregnancy. Eating a fertility diet can also help to increase the chances of a successful implantation of the embryo, which is the first step in the conception process. Eating a fertility diet can also help to increase the chances of a successful conception, as the body will be more receptive to the embryo.

Eating a fertility diet can also help to reduce the risk of certain complications during pregnancy. Eating a fertility diet can help to provide the body with the essential nutrients needed to support a healthy pregnancy. Eating a fertility diet can also help to reduce the risk of certain pregnancy complications such as preterm labor and preeclampsia. Eating a fertility diet can also help to reduce the risk of certain birth defects, such as neural tube defects.

Eating a fertility diet can also help to reduce the risk of certain reproductive issues. Eating a fertility diet can help to reduce the risk of certain reproductive issues such as endometriosis and PCOS. Eating a fertility diet can also help to reduce the risk of certain reproductive cancers, such as ovarian and uterine cancer.

Eating a fertility diet can also help to reduce the risk of certain lifestyle issues. Eating a fertility diet can help to reduce the risk of certain lifestyle issues such as stress, depression, and anxiety. Eating a fertility diet can also help to reduce the risk of certain unhealthy habits, such as smoking and excessive alcohol consumption.

In conclusion, eating a fertility diet can provide many benefits to women, ranging from improved overall health and fertility to increased chances of conception. Eating a fertility diet can help to create a healthy and balanced environment in the body to support conception and a healthy pregnancy. Eating a fertility diet can also help to reduce the risk of certain diseases and conditions, reproductive issues and lifestyle issues. Eating a fertility diet is an essential part of any woman's fertility plan and is an important step in becoming a mother.

CHAPTER 3

Foods to Avoid in Order to Conceive

When trying to conceive, many couples are willing to try anything in order to increase their chances of success. However, one of the most important, yet often overlooked, aspects of trying to conceive is diet. Eating certain foods can have a significant impact on fertility, so it is important to be aware of which foods to avoid in order to maximize your chances of conception.

1. High-Fat Foods: High-fat foods, such as fast food, fried foods, and processed meats, can negatively impact fertility because they contain saturated and trans fats, which can lead to weight gain and insulin resistance. Studies have found that a high-fat diet can reduce fertility in both men and women, so it is important to limit your intake of these types of foods.

2. Alcohol: While an occasional glass of wine is likely not going to have an effect on your fertility, heavy drinking can have a negative impact. Studies have found that drinking more than two alcoholic beverages per day can reduce fertility in men, while women who drink heavily can have difficulty with ovulation. Therefore, it is best to limit your intake of alcohol when trying to conceive.

3. Caffeine: Caffeine has been linked to decreased fertility in both men and women.

Studies have found that women who consume more than 300mg of caffeine per day have a lower chance of conceiving, while men who consume more than 500mg of caffeine per day have a lower sperm count. Therefore, it is best to limit your intake of caffeine when trying to get pregnant.

4. Sugar: Consuming too much sugar can lead to weight gain, which can have a negative effect on fertility. Studies have found that women who are overweight or obese have a higher risk of infertility, so it is important to limit your intake of sugary foods and drinks.

5. Processed Foods: Processed foods, such as chips, crackers, and other snacks, are usually high in fat, sugar, and sodium, which can all have a negative impact on fertility. In addition, these types of foods are usually low in essential nutrients, such as protein and fiber, which are important for fertility. Therefore, it is best to limit your intake of processed foods when trying to conceive.

6. High-Mercury Fish: Fish is an excellent source of protein and essential fatty acids, which are important for fertility. However, some types of fish, such as tuna, swordfish, and mackerel, are high in mercury, which can have a negative effect on fertility. Therefore, it is best to limit your intake of these types of fish when trying to conceive.

7. Deli Meats: Deli meats, such as ham, bologna, and salami, are often processed and high in sodium, which can have a negative effect on fertility. In addition, these types of meats can also be high in nitrates, which can have a detrimental effect on sperm quality. Therefore, it is best to limit your intake of deli meats when trying to conceive.

These are just a few of the foods to avoid when trying to conceive. Eating a healthy diet is important for fertility, so it is important to be mindful of what you are putting into your body. By avoiding the foods listed above, you can increase your chances of conceiving and have a healthy pregnancy.

Foods to Eat in Order to Conceive

When trying to conceive, diet plays an important role in a couple's success. Eating the right foods can help improve fertility, increase the chances of conception, and promote overall health. There are a variety of fertility-friendly foods that can help a couple conceive.

1. Antioxidants are key in helping to improve fertility. These are found in a variety of foods, including fruits and vegetables. For instance, blueberries and strawberries are packed with antioxidants and can help improve fertility. Other antioxidant-rich foods include apples, oranges, spinach, and kale. Eating these foods can help reduce inflammation and protect sperm from harmful free radicals, helping to improve the chances of conception.

2. Folic acid is also important for fertility. This nutrient helps the body produce healthy eggs and sperm, and is found in several foods. Leafy green vegetables such as spinach, broccoli, and kale are packed with folic acid. Other sources of folic acid include fortified breakfast cereals and breads, nuts, legumes, and fortified orange juice.

3. Omega-3 fatty acids are also essential for fertility. These fats are found in fatty fish such as salmon, tuna, mackerel, and herring. They are also found in walnuts, flaxseed, and chia seeds. Eating foods rich in omega-3 fatty acids can help improve the quality of the eggs and sperm, increasing the chances of conception.

4. Couples should also consider eating more complex carbohydrates. Complex carbohydrates are found in whole grain breads, pastas, and cereals. They are also found in beans, lentils, and quinoa. Eating these foods can help to stabilize blood sugar levels, which can help to improve fertility.

5. Eggs are another important food to eat when trying to conceive. Eggs are an excellent source of protein and are packed with essential vitamins and minerals. Eating a few eggs a day can help to improve fertility and increase the chances of conception.

In addition to eating fertility-friendly foods, couples should also consider making lifestyle changes to improve fertility. Smoking, drinking, and taking certain medications can all have a negative impact on fertility. If either partner is taking any medications, it is important to speak to a doctor or fertility specialist to ensure they are safe to take while trying to conceive.

Making dietary and lifestyle changes can help to improve fertility and increase the chances of conception. Eating a variety of fertility-friendly foods such as fruits and vegetables, complex carbohydrates, and omega-3 fatty acids can help to improve egg and sperm quality. Additionally, avoiding smoking, drinking, and certain medications can help to improve fertility. Incorporating these dietary and lifestyle changes can help a couple achieve their goal of having a baby.

PART 2:
Recipes to Reduce Inflammation and Balance Hormones

CHAPTER 4

Anti-inflammation Meal Plan

Day 1:

Breakfast: Overnight Oats with Blueberries And Chia Seeds.

Ingredients:

- -1/2 cup oats
- -1/2 cup almond milk
- -2 tablespoons chia seeds
- -1/2 cup blueberries (fresh or frozen)
- -1 teaspoon honey (optional)
- -1/4 teaspoon vanilla extract

Directions:

- In a medium bowl, combine oats, almond milk, chia seeds, honey, and vanilla extract.
- Stir until all ingredients are combined.
- Add blueberries and mix until evenly distributed.
- Cover the bowl and place in the fridge overnight.
- In the morning, remove from the fridge and enjoy.
- You can top the oats with your favorite toppings such as nuts, fruit, or a drizzle of honey.
- Enjoy!

Lunch: Quinoa and Vegetable Stir-Fry

Ingredients:

- -1 cup quinoa
- -1 tablespoon olive oil
- -1 onion, diced
- -1 red bell pepper, diced
- -1 cup mushrooms, sliced
- -1 cup broccoli florets
- -1/2 cup frozen corn
- -1 teaspoon garlic powder
- -1 teaspoon onion powder
- -1 teaspoon ground cumin
- -1/2 teaspoon chili powder
- -Salt and pepper, to taste
- -1/4 cup soy sauce

Instructions:

- Prepare the quinoa as directed on the package.
- Heat the olive oil in a sizable skillet or wok over medium-high heat.
- Add the diced onion and sauté for 3-4 minutes, until it begins to soften.
- Add the bell pepper, mushrooms, and broccoli and cook for an additional 3-4 minutes.
- Add the frozen corn and the seasonings, and cook for 1-2 minutes.
- Add the cooked quinoa and the soy sauce and stir to combine.
- Cook for an additional 1-2 minutes until everything is heated through.

- Serve warm. Enjoy!

Dinner: Baked Salmon with Roasted Asparagus

Ingredients:
- 2 salmon fillets
- 2 cloves of garlic, minced
- 2 tablespoons olive oil
- 2 tablespoons lemon juice
- Salt and pepper to taste
- 1 bunch of asparagus
- 2 tablespoons butter
- 1 tablespoon of chopped fresh parsley

Instructions:
1. Preheat oven to 400°F.
2. Place salmon fillets on a baking sheet lined with parchment paper.
3. In a small bowl, mix together the garlic, olive oil, lemon juice, salt and pepper.
4. Brush the mixture over the salmon.
5. Place the asparagus on the same baking sheet, and drizzle with the butter.
6. Bake in preheated oven for 20 minutes.
7. Sprinkle with chopped fresh parsley and enjoy!

Day 2:

Breakfast: Smoothie Bowl with Banana, Almond Milk, and Spinach

Ingredients:

- 1 banana
- 1 cup almond milk
- 1 cup spinach

Instructions:

1. Peel the banana and cut into slices.
2. Place the banana slices in a blender.
3. Add the almond milk and spinach to the blender.
4. Blend until smooth and creamy.
5. Pour the smoothie into a bowl.
6. Top with desired toppings such as granola, chia seeds, and fresh fruit. Enjoy!

Lunch: Kale Salad with Tempeh and Avocado

Ingredients:

- 2 bunches kale, chopped
- 1 package tempeh, cooked and cubed
- 1 avocado, diced
- 2 tablespoons olive oil
- 2 tablespoons apple cider vinegar
- 1 teaspoon honey
- 1 teaspoon Dijon mustard
- Salt and pepper, to taste

Instructions:

- In a large bowl, combine the chopped kale and tempeh.
- In a separate small bowl, whisk together the olive oil, apple cider vinegar, honey, and Dijon mustard.
- Pour the dressing over the kale and tempeh and toss to combine.
- Add the diced avocado and toss again.
- To taste, add salt and pepper to the food.
- Serve and enjoy!

Dinner: Grilled Vegetable Wrap with Hummus

Ingredients:

- 2 tablespoons olive oil
- 1 red pepper, sliced
- 1 yellow pepper, sliced
- 1/2 red onion, sliced
- 1/2 cup mushrooms, sliced
- 1 teaspoon garlic powder
- 1/4 teaspoon salt
- 1/4 teaspoon pepper
- 4 whole wheat wraps
- 1/2 cup prepared hummus
- 4 leaves lettuce

Instructions:

1. Preheat grill or grill pan to medium-high heat.
2. In a large bowl, combine the olive oil, peppers, onion, mushrooms, garlic powder, salt and pepper. Toss to combine.

3. Place the vegetables on the grill and cook until they are tender and lightly charred, stirring occasionally, about 8 minutes.
4. Remove the vegetables from the heat and let cool slightly.
5. Place each wrap on a plate. Each wrap should have 2 tablespoons of hummus on it.
6. Top each wrap with a lettuce leaf and a quarter of the grilled vegetables.
7. Fold the wrap and serve. Enjoy!

Day 3:

Breakfast: Almond Butter Toast with Banana Slices

Ingredients:

- 2 pieces of multigrain or whole wheat bread
- 2 tablespoons of almond butter
- 1 banana, sliced
- Pinch of ground cinnamon
- Honey (optional)

Instructions:

1. Toast the two slices of bread in a toaster or on a skillet.
2. Spread the almond butter on the toast slices.
3. Arrange the sliced banana over the almond butter.
4. Sprinkle the ground cinnamon over the banana slices.
5. Drizzle with honey, if desired.
6. Serve and enjoy!

Lunch: Chickpea and Vegetable Soup

Ingredients:

- 2 tablespoons olive oil
- 1 onion, diced
- 2 cloves garlic, minced
- 1 large carrot, diced
- 1 large potato, diced
- 1 red bell pepper, diced
- 3 cups vegetable broth
- 1 can (14.5 ounces) diced tomatoes
- 1 can (15 ounces) washed and drained chickpeas
- 1 teaspoon dried oregano
- 1 teaspoon dried thyme
- 1 teaspoon paprika
- Salt and pepper, to taste

Instructions:

1. In a sizable soup pot set over medium heat, warm the olive oil.
2. Add the onion and garlic, and cook for about 4 minutes, until the onion is softened and translucent.
3. Add the carrot, potato, and bell pepper, and cook for another 5 minutes.
4. Add the vegetable broth, diced tomatoes, chickpeas, oregano, thyme, and paprika.
5. Bring to a boil, reduce heat to low, and simmer for 20-30 minutes, until the vegetables are tender.
6. Taste and, if necessary, add additional salt and pepper to the seasoning.
7. Serve hot. Enjoy!

Dinner: Roasted Sweet Potato and Black Bean Tacos

Ingredients:

- -2 sweet potatoes, peeled and cut into 1/2-inch cubes
- -1/4 cup olive oil
- -1 teaspoon chili powder
- -1/2 teaspoon cumin
- -1/4 teaspoon garlic powder
- -1/4 teaspoon smoked paprika
- -1/4 teaspoon salt
- -1 15-ounce can black beans, drained and rinsed
- -1/2 cup corn
- -1/4 cup diced red onion
- -1/4 cup chopped cilantro
- -8 small flour tortillas
- -1/2 cup guacamole
- -1/2 cup shredded cheese
- -1/2 cup salsa

Instructions:

1. Set the oven's temperature to 375 degrees Fahrenheit.
2. Place the sweet potatoes on a baking sheet, then drizzle with olive oil and sprinkle with chili powder, cumin, garlic powder, smoked paprika, and salt. Toss the potatoes until they are evenly coated in the seasoning.
3. Roast the potatoes in the oven for 25-30 minutes, or until they are tender and golden.
4. In a medium bowl, combine the black beans, corn, red onion, and cilantro.
5. Heat the tortillas in a large skillet over medium heat.

6. To assemble the tacos, spoon some of the sweet potato mixture onto each tortilla, then top with the black bean mixture, guacamole, cheese, and salsa.
7. Serve the tacos warm. Enjoy!

Day 4:

Breakfast: Avocado Toast with Feta Cheese

Ingredients:

- -2 slices of whole-wheat bread
- -1/2 a ripe avocado
- -1/4 cup crumbled feta cheese
- -1 tablespoon olive oil
- -1 teaspoon lemon juice
- -Salt and pepper to taste

Instructions:

1. Toast the bread until lightly golden and crispy.
2. Cut the avocado in half, remove the seed, and scoop the flesh into a bowl.
3. Mash the avocado with a fork until smooth.
4. Add the feta cheese, olive oil, and lemon juice to the mashed avocado and mix until combined.
5. Spread the avocado mixture on the toasted bread slices.
6. Season to taste with salt and pepper.
7. Serve and enjoy!

Lunch: Quinoa Bowl with Roasted Vegetables

Ingredients:

- -1 cup quinoa
- -1 red pepper, chopped
- -1 zucchini, chopped
- -1 red onion, chopped
- -2 cloves garlic, minced
- -2 tablespoons olive oil
- -2 tablespoons balsamic vinegar
- -1 teaspoon dried oregano
- -Salt and pepper to taste
- -1 cup cooked black beans
- -1/4 cup crumbled feta cheese

Instructions:

1. Preheat oven to 400 degrees F.
2. In a bowl, combine quinoa, red pepper, zucchini, red onion, garlic, olive oil, balsamic vinegar, oregano, salt, and pepper. Stir until everything is well combined.
3. Spread the quinoa mixture onto a baking sheet.
4. Bake in the oven for 20 minutes until vegetables are tender and lightly browned.
5. While the vegetables are baking, cook the black beans according to package instructions.
6. Divide the roasted vegetables and cooked beans into 4 bowls.
7. Top each bowl with feta cheese.
8. Serve and enjoy!

Dinner: Baked Cod with Steamed Broccoli

Ingredients:

- -2 pieces of cod
- -2 tablespoons of olive oil
- -1/2 teaspoon of garlic powder
- -1/4 teaspoon of paprika
- -1/4 teaspoon of dried parsley
- -1/4 teaspoon of salt
- -1/4 teaspoon of black pepper
- -1 head of broccoli

Instructions:

1. Preheat oven to 400 degrees F.

2. Place cod pieces on a baking sheet lined with parchment paper.

3. Rub olive oil all over the cod pieces.

4. Sprinkle garlic powder, paprika, parsley, salt and pepper over the cod.

5. Bake cod in preheated oven for 15-20 minutes or until cod is cooked through.

6. Meanwhile, fill a pot halfway with water and bring to a boil.

7. Cut broccoli into smaller florets and add to boiling water.

8. Reduce heat and simmer for 3-4 minutes or until broccoli is tender.

9. Drain broccoli and serve with baked cod. Enjoy!

Day 5:

Breakfast: Omelet with bell peppers, mushrooms, and spinach

Ingredients:

- -3 large eggs
- -1/4 cup of diced bell peppers
- -1/4 cup of diced mushrooms
- -1/4 cup of spinach
- -Salt and pepper to taste
- -1 tablespoon of butter

Instructions:

1. In a bowl, whisk together eggs, bell peppers, mushrooms, spinach, salt, and pepper.
2. Heat a small non-stick skillet over medium-high heat and add butter.
3. Once the butter has melted, add the egg and vegetable mixture and spread evenly across the pan.
4. Cook for about 3 minutes until the edges of the omelet have set and the bottom is lightly golden.
5. Flip the omelet and cook for another 2 minutes until the center is cooked through.
6. Serve the omelet hot topped with your favorite toppings. Enjoy!

Lunch: Lentil and Vegetable Salad

Ingredients:

- 1 cup green lentils

- 2 cups chopped vegetables (such as carrots, celery, bell peppers, tomatoes, onions, etc.)
- 2 tablespoons olive oil
- 2 tablespoons lemon juice
- 2 tablespoons chopped fresh herbs (such as parsley, oregano, thyme, etc.)
- 1 teaspoon salt
- 1/4 teaspoon black pepper

Instructions:

1. Rinse the lentils in cold water and place in a large pot. Bring to a boil while being covered with 2 inches of water. Lentils should be cooked for 15 to 20 minutes over low heat.
2. In a large bowl, combine chopped vegetables, olive oil, lemon juice, fresh herbs, salt, and pepper.
3. Add the cooked lentils to the bowl and toss to combine.
4. Refrigerate for at least 1 hour before serving. Enjoy!

Dinner: Grilled Tempeh with Brown Rice and Sautéed Kale

Ingredients:

- 4 ounces tempeh, cut into thin strips
- 1/2 cup cooked brown rice
- 1/2 cup kale, roughly chopped
- 2 tablespoons olive oil
- 1 teaspoon garlic powder
- Salt and pepper, to taste

Instructions:

1. Start your grill or grill pan by heating it to medium-high.
2. Place the tempeh strips on the grill and cook for 3-4 minutes per side, or until they are golden brown and slightly charred.
3. In a separate pan over medium heat, heat the olive oil.
4. Once the oil is hot, add the kale and sauté for about 3 minutes, or until the kale is wilted and lightly browned.
5. Add the cooked brown rice, garlic powder, salt and pepper, and stir to combine.
6. Cook for an additional 1-2 minutes, or until the rice is heated through.
7. Serve the tempeh with the sautéed kale and brown rice. Enjoy!

Day 6:

Breakfast: Acai Bowl with Banana And Almond Butter

Ingredients:

- 1/2 cup frozen Acai puree
- 1/2 banana, sliced
- 1/4 cup almond butter
- 2 tablespoons honey
- 1/4 cup almond milk
- 1/4 cup rolled oats
- 1/4 cup granola
- 1/4 cup fresh berries

Instructions:

1. Place the Acai puree, banana, almond butter, honey, and almond milk in a blender and blend until smooth.
2. Pour the Acai mixture into a bowl and top with the rolled oats, granola, and fresh berries.
3. Serve the Acai bowl with banana and almond butter immediately. Enjoy!

Lunch: Roasted Vegetable Wrap with Hummus

Ingredients:

- 1 red bell pepper, chopped
- 1 yellow bell pepper, chopped
- 1 zucchini, chopped
- ½ red onion, chopped
- 2 cloves of garlic, minced
- 2 tablespoons olive oil
- Salt and pepper to taste
- 4 whole wheat wraps
- Hummus
- Fresh greens like spinach or arugula

Instructions:

1. Preheat oven to 400°F (205°C).
2. In a mixing bowl, combine the chopped peppers, zucchini, red onion, garlic, olive oil, salt, and pepper. Toss to combine.
3. Spread the vegetables out on a baking sheet and bake for 25 minutes, stirring halfway through baking.
4. Once the vegetables are done baking, let them cool for a few minutes before assembling the wraps.

5. To assemble the wraps, spread a generous amount of hummus onto each wrap.
6. Top with fresh greens, and roasted vegetables.
7. Roll up the wraps, cut in half, and enjoy!

Dinner: Baked Salmon with Roasted Brussels Sprouts

Ingredients:

- 1 lb. salmon fillet
- 2 cups Brussels sprouts
- 2 cloves garlic, minced
- 2 tablespoons olive oil
- Salt and pepper to taste
- 2 tablespoons lemon juice
- 2 tablespoons butter
- 2 tablespoons chopped fresh parsley

Instructions:

1. Preheat oven to 400 degrees F.
2. Place salmon fillet on a lightly greased baking sheet.
3. In a medium bowl, combine Brussels sprouts, garlic, olive oil, salt, and pepper. Toss to coat.
4. Spread Brussels sprouts onto the baking sheet around the salmon.
5. Drizzle lemon juice and butter over the salmon and Brussels sprouts.
6. Bake for 15 minutes or until salmon is cooked through and Brussels sprouts are tender.
7. Sprinkle with chopped fresh parsley before serving. Enjoy!

Day 7:

Breakfast: Smoothie Bowl with Banana, Almond Milk, And Spinach

Ingredients:

- -1 banana
- -1 cup of almond milk
- -2 cups of spinach
- -Toppings of your choice (e.g., chia seeds, nuts, shredded coconut, fresh fruit, etc.)

Directions:

1. Slice the banana after peeling it.
2. Place the banana slices, almond milk, and spinach in a blender.
3. Blend until smooth.
4. Pour the smoothie into a bowl.
5. Top with your favorite toppings.
6. Enjoy!

Lunch: Quinoa and Black Bean Bowl With Avocado

Ingredients:

- -1 cup uncooked quinoa
- -1 15-ounce can of rinsed and drained black beans
- -1 tbsp olive oil
- -1 tsp cumin
- -1/4 tsp cayenne pepper
- -1/2 tsp paprika
- -Salt and pepper to taste

- -1/2 cup diced tomatoes
- -1/2 cup diced red onion
- -1/4 cup chopped cilantro
- -1 ripe avocado, diced
- -Juice of 1 lime

Instructions:

1. Prepare the quinoa as directed on the package.
2. Add the olive oil to a big skillet that is already hot over medium heat.
3. Add the black beans and spices and cook for 5 minutes, stirring occasionally.
4. Add the tomatoes, red onion, and cilantro and cook for an additional 2 minutes.
5. In a large bowl, combine the cooked quinoa and black bean mixture.
6. Add the diced avocado and lime juice and stir to combine.
7. Serve warm or cold. Enjoy!

Dinner: Grilled Veggie Kebabs with Quinoa

Ingredients:

- -1 cup of cooked quinoa
- -1 red bell pepper, diced into 1-inch pieces.
- -1 yellow bell pepper, cut into 1 inch cubes
- -1 zucchini, cut into 1 inch cubes
- -1 red onion, cut into 1 inch cubes
- -1 portobello mushroom, diced into 1-inch pieces.

- -1 tablespoon olive oil
- -Salt and pepper to taste

Instructions:

1. Preheat your outdoor grill or indoor grill pan to medium-high heat.
2. In a large bowl, combine the cooked quinoa, bell peppers, zucchini, onion, and mushroom. Drizzle with olive oil, and season with salt and pepper, to taste.
3. Carefully thread the vegetables onto skewers.
4. Grill the kebabs on both sides until lightly charred and tender, about 8-10 minutes.
5. Serve the kebabs with the cooked quinoa and enjoy!

CHAPTER 5

Hormone Balancing Diet Meal Plan

Day 1

Breakfast: Two poached eggs with spinach and feta on a whole grain toast

Ingredients:

- 2 eggs
- 2 slices of whole grain bread
- 2 handfuls of spinach
- 2 tablespoons of feta cheese
- 2 tablespoons of butter
- 1 tablespoon of white vinegar
- Salt and pepper to taste

Instructions:

1. Start by bringing some water to a boil in a pot.
2. Once boiling, reduce the heat to a gentle simmer and add the white vinegar to the water.
3. Crack each egg into a separate small bowl and carefully pour the eggs into the water, one at a time.
4. Allow the eggs to poach for about 4 minutes, or until the whites are set and the yolks are still runny.
5. Meanwhile, melt the butter in a skillet over medium heat.
6. Add the spinach and sauté until wilted, about 1-2 minutes.

7. Toast the bread until golden brown.
8. To assemble, place one slice of toast on each plate and top each with the wilted spinach.
9. Carefully remove the poached eggs from the water with a slotted spoon and place one egg on each slice of toast.
10. Sprinkle each egg with feta cheese and season with salt and pepper to taste.
11. Serve warm and enjoy!

Lunch: Lentil and vegetable soup with a side salad

Lentil and Vegetable Soup

Ingredients:

- 2 tablespoons of olive oil
- 1 onion, chopped
- 2 cloves of garlic, minced
- 2 carrots, chopped
- 2 celery stalks, chopped
- 2 potatoes, chopped
- 1 teaspoon of cumin
- 1 teaspoon of coriander
- ½ teaspoon of turmeric
- ¼ teaspoon of cayenne pepper
- 4 cups of vegetable broth
- 1 cup of green lentils, rinsed
- 1 can of diced tomatoes
- Salt and pepper to taste

Instructions:

1. In a big pot over medium heat, warm the olive oil.
2. Add the onion, garlic, carrots, celery, and potatoes. Cook for 5 minutes, stirring occasionally.
3. Add the cayenne, turmeric, cumin, and coriander. Cook for 1 minute, stirring constantly.
4. Add the vegetable broth and lentils. Bring to a boil, then reduce the heat and simmer for 20 minutes.
5. Add the diced tomatoes and simmer for 10 minutes.
6. Taste and adjust the seasoning with salt and pepper, if needed.
7. Serve with a side salad. Enjoy!

Side Salad

Ingredients:

- 4 cups of mixed greens
- ½ cup of cherry tomatoes, halved
- ½ cup of sliced cucumbers
- ¼ cup of diced red onion
- ¼ cup of crumbled feta cheese
- 2 tablespoons of olive oil
- 1 tablespoon of lemon juice
- 1 teaspoon of honey
- Salt and pepper to taste

Instructions:

1. In a large bowl, combine the mixed greens, cherry tomatoes, cucumbers, red onion, and feta cheese.
2. In a small bowl, whisk together the olive oil, lemon juice, honey, and salt and pepper.
3. Drizzle the dressing over the salad and toss to combine.

4. Serve alongside the lentil and vegetable soup. Enjoy!

Dinner: Salmon on the grill with roasted vegetables and quinoa

Ingredients:

- 2 salmon filets
- 2 cups cooked quinoa
- 2 cups diced vegetables of your choice (e.g. bell peppers, zucchini, onions, mushrooms)
- 2 tablespoons olive oil
- Salt and pepper to taste
- Fresh herbs of your choice (e.g. thyme, rosemary, oregano)

Instructions:

1. Preheat the oven to 400°F.
2. Place the vegetables on a baking sheet and drizzle with olive oil, salt, and pepper.
3. Roast the vegetables for 20 minutes, or until they are tender.
4. Meanwhile, season the salmon with salt and pepper and any fresh herbs of your choice.
5. Heat a non-stick skillet over medium-high heat and add the salmon.
6. Cook the salmon for 4-5 minutes per side, or until cooked through.
7. Serve the salmon with the roasted vegetables and quinoa.
8. Enjoy!

Snack: Fresh fruit and nut butter

Ingredients:

- -1 cup of fresh, seasonal fruit (such as apples, bananas, strawberries, or blueberries)
- -2 tablespoons of nut butter (such as almond, peanut, or cashew)
- -1 teaspoon of honey (optional)

Instructions:

1. Wash and prepare the fruit. Slice or dice the fruit into small, bite-sized pieces.
2. Place the prepared fruit into a bowl.
3. Add the nut butter and honey to the bowl and mix until evenly combined.
4. Serve and enjoy!

Day 2

Breakfast: Overnight oats with almond milk, fruit, and chia seeds.

Ingredients

- -1/2 cup rolled oats
- -1/2 cup almond milk
- -1/2 tablespoon chia seeds
- -1/4 cup mixed berries (fresh or frozen)

Instructions

1. In a medium bowl, combine oats, almond milk and chia seeds. All the ingredients should be thoroughly mixed.

2. Add mixed berries and stir until evenly distributed.
3. Cover the bowl and refrigerate overnight.
4. In the morning, remove from the refrigerator and enjoy!

Lunch: Arugula salad with grilled chicken and avocado

Ingredients:

- -1 lb boneless, skinless chicken breasts
- -2 avocados, diced
- -2 cups arugula
- -1/4 cup olive oil
- -2 tablespoons fresh lemon juice
- -1 tablespoon honey
- -1 teaspoon sea salt
- -1/2 teaspoon freshly ground black pepper
- -1/4 cup crumbled feta cheese

Instructions:

1. Preheat grill to medium-high heat.
2. Grill chicken for 4 to 5 minutes per side, until cooked through. Before slicing, remove from heat and allow it cool for five minutes.
3. In a large bowl, combine arugula, olive oil, lemon juice, honey, salt, and pepper. Gently toss to combine.
4. Add in the chicken, diced avocados, and feta cheese. Gently toss to combine.
5. Serve immediately. Enjoy!

Dinner: Baked sweet potato with black beans and steamed vegetables

Ingredients:

- 2 sweet potatoes
- ½ cup cooked black beans
- ½ cup steamed vegetables of choice
- 2 tablespoons olive oil
- 2 tablespoons chopped fresh herbs (parsley, oregano, thyme, etc.)
- Salt and pepper, to taste
- 1 tablespoon fresh lemon juice (optional)

Instructions

1. Preheat oven to 400°F.
2. Scrub sweet potatoes clean, then pierce with a fork several times. Bake for 40 minutes, or until tender, on a baking sheet.
3. Meanwhile, steam vegetables according to package instructions.
4. Once sweet potatoes are done, remove from oven and let cool for 5 minutes.
5. Cut each sweet potato lengthwise and carefully scoop out the flesh into a medium-sized bowl.
6. Add black beans, steamed vegetables, olive oil, herbs, salt, and pepper to the bowl. Mix until everything is well combined.
7. Divide the mixture evenly between the two sweet potato skins.
8. Place stuffed sweet potatoes on a baking sheet and bake for an additional 10 minutes.
9. Drizzle with lemon juice, if desired, and serve. Enjoy!

Snack: Greek yogurt with honey and walnuts

Ingredients:

- -2 cups Greek yogurt
- -2 tablespoons honey
- -1/4 cup chopped walnuts

Instructions:

1. In a medium bowl, combine the Greek yogurt and honey.
2. Stir until the honey is fully incorporated into the yogurt.
3. Add the chopped walnuts and stir to combine.
4. Serve in individual bowls or as a dip with fresh fruit. Enjoy!

Day 3

Breakfast: Smoothie bowl with banana, almond milk, almond butter, and cacao powder

Ingredients:

- -1 large banana
- -1 cup of almond milk
- -2 tablespoons of almond butter
- -2 tablespoons of cacao powder

Instructions:

1. Peel and slice the banana into small chunks.
2. Place the banana chunks into a blender.
3. Add 1 cup of almond milk to the blender.

4. Blend the ingredients until smooth.
5. Pour the mixture into a bowl.
6. Drizzle 2 tablespoons of almond butter over the top.
7. Sprinkle 2 tablespoons of cacao powder over the top.
8. Serve your smoothie bowl and enjoy!

Lunch: Quinoa bowl with roasted vegetables and chickpeas

Ingredients:

- -2 cups cooked quinoa
- -1 cup uncooked chickpeas
- -2 cups mixed vegetables (such as broccoli, bell peppers, zucchini, etc.)
- -2 tablespoons olive oil
- -Salt and pepper to taste
- -1/4 cup crumbled feta cheese (optional)
- -2 tablespoons chopped fresh parsley (optional)

Instructions:

1. Preheat oven to 375°F.
2. Spread the chickpeas and vegetables on a large baking sheet. Season with salt and pepper and drizzle olive oil on top.
3. Roast for 25 minutes, stirring occasionally, until the vegetables are tender and lightly browned.
4. Divide the quinoa among four bowls. Top each bowl with equal amounts of roasted vegetables and chickpeas.
5. Sprinkle feta cheese and parsley over the top, if desired.
6. Serve warm. Enjoy!

Dinner: Grilled chicken with wild rice and grilled asparagus

Ingredients:

- 4 boneless chicken breasts
- 2 tablespoons olive oil
- 1 teaspoon garlic powder
- 1 teaspoon onion powder
- 1 teaspoon paprika
- 1 teaspoon black pepper
- 1 teaspoon sea salt
- 2 cups cooked wild rice
- 1 bunch of asparagus, trimmed
- 2 tablespoons butter

Instructions:

1. Preheat the grill to medium heat.
2. In a small bowl, combine the olive oil, garlic powder, onion powder, paprika, black pepper, and sea salt.
3. Rub the mixture onto the chicken breasts and place on the preheated grill. Cook for 6-7 minutes on each side, or until the chicken is cooked through.
4. In the interim, make the wild rice as directed on the package.
5. Toss the asparagus in the butter, and then place on the grill. Cook for 2-3 minutes on each side, or until the asparagus is tender.
6. Serve the grilled chicken with the wild rice and grilled asparagus. Enjoy!

Snack: Apple slices with almond butter

Ingredients:

- -2 large apples
- -½ cup creamy almond butter
- -2 tablespoons honey
- -1 teaspoon ground cinnamon
- -1 teaspoon ground nutmeg

Instructions:

1. Preheat the oven to 350°F.
2. Slice the apples into ½-inch thick slices.
3. Place the apple slices on a parchment-lined baking sheet.
4. In a small bowl, mix together the almond butter, honey, cinnamon and nutmeg.
5. Spread the almond butter mixture on top of each apple slice.
6. Bake in the preheated oven for 15 minutes, or until the apples are tender.
7. Serve warm and enjoy!

Day 4

Breakfast: Egg muffins with bell peppers and kale

Ingredients:

- 8 large eggs
- 1/4 cup diced bell peppers
- 1/4 cup diced kale
- Salt and pepper to taste
- Cooking spray

Instructions:

1. Preheat oven to 350°F.
2. Grease a 12-cup muffin tin with cooking spray and set aside.
3. In a medium bowl, whisk together eggs, bell peppers, kale, salt, and pepper until well combined.
4. Divide the egg mixture evenly among the muffin cups.
5. Bake for 20-25 minutes, or until the egg muffins are set and golden brown.
6. Let to cool completely before serving. Enjoy!

Lunch: Hummus wrap with cucumber and tomato

Ingredients:

- -2 whole wheat tortillas
- 1/2 cup prepared hummus
- 1/2 cup diced cucumber
- 1/2 cup diced tomatoes
- 1/4 cup shredded lettuce

Instructions:

1. Spread a thin layer of hummus on each tortilla.
2. Top with cucumber, tomatoes, and lettuce.
3. Roll up each tortilla tightly.
4. To serve, cut each wrap in half.

Dinner: Roasted Brussels sprouts, baked salmon, and sweet potatoes.

Ingredients:

- 1 pound Salmon fillet, skinless
- 1 pound Brussels sprouts, halved
- 1 large sweet potato, peeled and cut into cubes
- 2 tablespoons olive oil
- 2 tablespoons lemon juice
- 2 cloves garlic, minced
- 1 teaspoon dried oregano
- 1 teaspoon dried thyme
- 1 teaspoon freshly ground black pepper
- Salt to taste

Instructions:

1. Preheat oven to 400°F.
2. Place the salmon fillet in an oven-safe dish and season with salt and pepper.
3. In a bowl, combine the Brussels sprouts, sweet potato, olive oil, lemon juice, garlic, oregano, thyme, and pepper. Toss to combine.
4. Place the Brussels sprouts and sweet potato mixture around the salmon in the dish.
5. Bake in the preheated oven for 20 minutes, or until the salmon is cooked through and the vegetables are tender.
6. Serve and enjoy!

Snack: Greek yogurt with granola and berries

Ingredients:

- 1/2 cup Greek yogurt
- 1/4 cup granola
- 1/4 cup mixed berries (blueberries, raspberries, blackberries, etc.)

Instructions:

1. In a bowl, spoon the Greek yogurt.
2. Sprinkle the granola over the yogurt.
3. Top the mixture with the mixed berries.
4. Enjoy!

Day 5

Breakfast: Avocado toast with an egg and a side of spinach

Avocado Toast with Egg and Spinach

Ingredients:

- 1 avocado
- 2 slices of whole grain bread
- 1 egg
- 1 teaspoon of olive oil
- Salt and pepper to taste
- 2 cups of baby spinach

Instructions:

1. A nonstick skillet is heated to medium-high heat

2. Cut the avocado into slices and spread it on the slices of bread.
3. Crack the egg into the skillet and cook until desired doneness.
4. Heat the olive oil in a separate skillet over medium heat. Baby spinach should be added and cooked until wilted.
5. Place the cooked egg on top of the avocado toast and season with salt and pepper.
6. Serve the avocado toast with the side of spinach. Enjoy!

Lunch: Grilled chicken salad with quinoa and feta

Ingredients:
- -2 boneless, skinless chicken breasts
- -1/2 cup cooked quinoa
- -1/3 cup crumbled feta cheese
- -1/4 cup diced red onion
- -2 tablespoons olive oil
- -1 tablespoon lemon juice
- -1 teaspoon dried oregano
- -Salt and pepper, to taste

Instructions:
1. Preheat an outdoor grill or indoor grill pan over medium-high heat.
2. Rub chicken breasts with 1 tablespoon of the olive oil and season with salt and pepper. Chicken should be cooked thoroughly on the grill for 5 to 7 minutes per side.
3. In a large bowl, combine quinoa, feta cheese, red onion, remaining olive oil, lemon juice, oregano, salt, and pepper.

4. Cut chicken into small cubes and add to quinoa mixture. Stir to combine.
5. Serve salad immediately, or chill in the refrigerator for up to 2 days. Enjoy!

Dinner: Vegetable stir-fry with brown rice

Ingredients:

- 2 tablespoons sesame oil
- 2 cloves garlic, minced
- 1 teaspoon fresh ginger, minced
- 1 onion, chopped
- 2 cups mixed vegetables, such as broccoli, carrots, bell pepper, mushrooms, and snow peas
- 3 tablespoons soy sauce
- 2 cups cooked brown rice

Instructions:

1. Heat the sesame oil in a wok or large skillet over medium-high heat.
2. After cooking for 1 minute, add the ginger and garlic.
3. After cooking for 2 minutes, add the onion.
4. Add the mixed vegetables and cook for 5 minutes, stirring frequently.
5. Add the soy sauce and stir to combine.
6. Add the cooked brown rice and stir to combine.
7. Cook for an additional 3-4 minutes, stirring occasionally, until the vegetables are tender and the rice is heated through.
8. Serve hot. Enjoy!

Snack: Trail mix with nuts and dried fruit

Ingredients:

- 1/2 cup of almonds
- 1/2 cup of walnuts
- 1/2 cup of cashews
- 1/2 cup of dried cranberries
- 1/2 cup of raisins
- 1/4 cup of sunflower seeds
- 1/4 cup of pumpkin seeds
- Optional: 1/4 cup of chocolate chips

Instructions:

1. Preheat the oven to 350°F.

2. Spread the almonds, walnuts, and cashews onto a baking sheet and roast in the preheated oven for 5-7 minutes, until lightly toasted.

3. Remove the baking sheet from the oven and let the nuts cool completely.

4. Place the cooled nuts in a large bowl and add the dried cranberries, raisins, sunflower seeds, and pumpkin seeds.

5. Mix the ingredients together until evenly distributed.

6. If desired, add the chocolate chips and mix them in.

7. Store the trail mix in an airtight container. Enjoy!

Day 6

Breakfast: Oatmeal with almond milk and nuts

Ingredients:

- -1 cup of rolled oats
- -1 cup of almond milk
- -2 tablespoons of maple syrup
- -2 tablespoons of chopped nuts (such as almonds, walnuts, or pecans)
- -1/4 teaspoon ground cinnamon
- -1/4 teaspoon of sea salt

Instructions:

1. In a small saucepan, bring the almond milk to a boil.

2. Stir in the rolled oats and reduce the heat to low. Cook for 3 minutes, stirring occasionally.

3. Add the maple syrup, chopped nuts, cinnamon and salt. Cook for an additional 2 minutes, stirring occasionally, until the oats are cooked through.

4. Serve the oatmeal hot, topped with additional chopped nuts, if desired. Enjoy!

Lunch: Baked sweet potato with black beans and steamed vegetables

Ingredients:

- 2 large sweet potatoes
- 1 can washed and drained black beans

- 1 cup of diced vegetables (such as bell peppers, carrots, and onions)
- 2 tablespoons olive oil
- 1 teaspoon ground cumin
- ½ teaspoon chili powder
- Salt and pepper to taste

Instructions:

1. Preheat oven to 400°F.
2. Cut sweet potatoes in half lengthwise, then slice into thin wedges. Place wedges on a greased baking sheet.
3. In a medium bowl, combine black beans, diced vegetables, olive oil, cumin, chili powder, salt, and pepper. Mix until all ingredients are combined.
4. Spread bean and vegetable mixture over the sweet potatoes.
5. Bake for 20 minutes, or until sweet potatoes are cooked through.
6. While the sweet potatoes are baking, steam the remaining vegetables in a steamer basket over boiling water for about 5 minutes, or until the vegetables are tender.
7. Serve the baked sweet potatoes with the steamed vegetables on the side. Enjoy!

Dinner: Salmon on the grill with roasted Brussels sprouts and quinoa

Ingredients:

- 4 (4 ounce) salmon fillets
- 2 tablespoons olive oil

- Salt and freshly ground black pepper
- 2 cups cooked quinoa
- 1 1/2 pounds of halved and trimmed Brussels sprouts
- 2 tablespoons melted butter
- 2 tablespoons freshly squeezed lemon juice
- 1 tablespoon minced garlic

Instructions:

1. Preheat the oven to 375°F (190°C).
2. Place the salmon fillets in a shallow baking dish. Add salt and pepper, then drizzle with the olive oil.
3. Spread the cooked quinoa in an even layer over the bottom of a large baking sheet. Place the Brussels sprouts on top of the quinoa. Drizzle with the melted butter, lemon juice, and garlic.
4. Roast the Brussels sprouts and quinoa in the preheated oven for 20 minutes, or until the Brussels sprouts are tender and lightly browned.
5. Meanwhile, heat an outdoor grill to medium-high heat. Place the salmon fillets on the grill and cook for 3 to 4 minutes per side, or until the salmon is cooked through.
6. Serve the grilled salmon with the roasted Brussels sprouts and quinoa. Enjoy!

Snack: Fresh fruit and nut butter

Ingredients:

- 2 cups of fresh fruit (ex. Strawberries, oranges, grapes, etc.)
- 2 tablespoons of nut butter (ex. Almond, cashew, peanut, etc.)

- 2 tablespoons of honey
- ½ teaspoon of cinnamon
- 2 tablespoons of shredded coconut (optional)

Instructions:

1. Cut the fruit into bite-sized pieces after washing.
2. Place the fruit in a bowl and set aside.
3. In a separate bowl, mix together the nut butter, honey, and cinnamon until well combined.
4. Pour the nut butter mixture over the fruit and gently mix until the fruit is evenly coated.
5. Sprinkle the shredded coconut over the top, if desired.
6. Serve the fruit and nut butter immediately and enjoy!

Day 7

Breakfast: Green smoothie with banana, spinach, almond milk, and almond butter

Ingredients:

- -1 banana
- -2 cups spinach
- -1 cup almond milk
- -2 tablespoons almond butter

Instructions:

1. Place the banana, spinach, almond milk, and almond butter in a blender.

2. Blend on high speed until the ingredients are well combined and the smoothie is creamy, about 2 minutes.
3. Pour the smoothie into a glass and enjoy!

Lunch: Arugula salad with grilled chicken and avocado

Ingredients:

- 2 boneless skinless chicken breasts
- 2 tablespoons olive oil
- Salt and pepper, to taste
- 4 cups arugula
- 1 avocado, diced
- 1/4 cup feta cheese, crumbled
- 2 tablespoons lemon juice
- 2 tablespoons olive oil

Instructions:

1. Preheat the grill to medium-high heat.
2. Rub the chicken with olive oil and season with salt and pepper.
3. Place the chicken on the preheated grill and cook for 5-7 minutes per side, or until the chicken is cooked through.
4. Remove the chicken from the grill and let it rest.
5. In a large bowl, combine the arugula, avocado, feta cheese, and lemon juice.
6. Slice up the chicken and mix it with the salad.
7. Drizzle with olive oil and toss to combine.
8. Serve and enjoy.

Dinner: Baked tofu with roasted vegetables and brown rice

Ingredients:

- -1 block extra-firm tofu, drained and pressed
- -1 red bell pepper, thinly sliced.
- -1 green bell pepper, cut into thin strips
- -1 small onion, thinly sliced
- -2 cloves garlic, minced
- -1/4 cup low-sodium soy sauce
- -1 tablespoon sesame oil
- -1/2 teaspoon ground ginger
- -1/4 teaspoon red pepper flakes
- -1 cup uncooked brown rice
- -2 cups vegetable broth
- -1 tablespoon olive oil

Instructions:

1. Preheat oven to 375 degrees F.
2. Place the pressed tofu on a parchment-lined baking sheet. Bake in preheated oven for 15 minutes.
3. In the meantime, preheat a big skillet to medium heat. Add olive oil and then add bell peppers, onion, and garlic. Sauté the vegetables for 5-7 minutes, or until they are soft.
4. In a small bowl, whisk together soy sauce, sesame oil, ground ginger, and red pepper flakes.
5. Once the tofu is done baking, remove from the oven and pour soy sauce mixture over the top. Use a spatula to gently toss the tofu in the mixture.
6. Place the tofu back on the baking sheet and bake for an additional 10 minutes.

7. While the tofu is baking, cook the rice according to package directions, using vegetable broth instead of water.
8. Once the tofu is done baking, remove from the oven and serve over cooked brown rice with roasted vegetables. Enjoy!

Snack: Greek yogurt with honey and walnuts

Ingredients:

- -2 cups of Greek yogurt
- -2 tablespoons of honey
- -1/4 cup of walnuts, chopped

Instructions:

1. In a medium bowl, mix together the Greek yogurt and honey until well combined.
2. Add the chopped walnuts and stir until they are evenly distributed throughout the yogurt.
3. Serve immediately, or chill in the fridge for 30 minutes before serving. Enjoy!

Part 3:

Boosting Fertility with Supplements and Herbs

CHAPTER 6

Supplements to Boost Fertility

Fertility is an important part of life and its health is paramount. Achieving a healthy pregnancy is the goal of many couples, and the proper use of supplements may help to increase fertility and improve the chances of conception. There are many supplements available on the market today that claim to boost fertility, and this article will discuss some of the supplements which may be helpful in increasing fertility. We will look at the types of supplements available and their potential benefits, as well as discussing the risks associated with taking supplements, and provide advice on how to choose the right supplements for you.

1. **Folic Acid:** Folic acid is an important supplement for boosting fertility as it helps to create and maintain healthy cells, including those of the reproductive system. Benefits include reducing the risk of neural tube defects in a developing baby, as well as potentially improving sperm quality. Risks include an increased risk of certain cancers in men, so it is important to discuss with your doctor before taking large doses.
2. **Coenzyme Q10 (CoQ10):** CoQ10 helps to improve egg and sperm quality, and has been known to increase fertility in both men and women. Benefits include improved egg quality and a greater chance of successful fertilization. Potential risks include nausea, vomiting and diarrhea if taken in high doses.

3. **Vitamin D:** Vitamin D is important for overall health and fertility, as it helps the body to absorb calcium and produce hormones. Benefits include improved egg and sperm quality, as well as increased chances of successful fertilization. Risks include vitamin D toxicity if taken in excessive amounts.
4. **Vitamin B12:** Vitamin B12 helps to improve egg and sperm quality, and is thought to increase the chance of successful implantation. Benefits include improved fertility, as well as improved energy levels. Risks include potential allergic reactions and interference with certain medications.
5. **Zinc:** Zinc is essential for healthy reproductive systems and helps to improve sperm quality. Benefits include improved egg and sperm quality, as well as increased chances of successful fertilization. Potential risks include nausea and vomiting if taken in high doses.
6. **L-Carnitine:** L-carnitine is an amino acid that helps improve sperm motility and quality. Benefits include improved sperm quality and motility, as well as increased chances of successful fertilization. Potential risks include nausea, vomiting and diarrhea if taken in high doses.
7. **Omega-3 Fatty Acids:** Omega-3 fatty acids are important for overall health and fertility, as they help to improve egg and sperm quality. Benefits include improved egg and sperm quality, as well as increased chances of successful fertilization. Potential risks include fishy burps and stomach upset.
8. **DHEA:** DHEA is a hormone that helps to improve egg and sperm quality, as well as increase the chance of successful implantation. Benefits include improved fertility, as well as increased energy levels.

Potential risks include acne, hair loss and interference with certain medications.

9. **Pycnogenol:** Pycnogenol is an antioxidant that helps to improve egg and sperm quality, as well as increase the chance of successful implantation. Benefits include improved egg and sperm quality, as well as increased chances of successful fertilization. Potential risks include nausea, vomiting and diarrhea if taken in high doses.
10. **Maca Root:** Maca root is a natural supplement that helps to improve egg and sperm quality, as well as increase the chance of successful implantation. Benefits include improved fertility, as well as increased energy levels. Potential risks include stomach upset and interference with certain medications.

CHAPTER 7

Herbal Remedies for Infertility

Herbal remedies for infertility have been used for centuries to help women become pregnant. Herbs have been used traditionally to help balance hormones, increase fertility, and support a healthy reproductive system.

The use of herbs is often a gentler, more natural way to treat infertility than drugs or surgery. While there is limited scientific evidence to support the effectiveness of herbal remedies for infertility, many women have found success in using them.

In this chapter, we will discuss the various herbs used for infertility, their possible benefits, and how to use them safely.

1. Red Clover: Red clover is a flowering plant that is high in phytoestrogens, lignans, and isoflavones. It has been used to treat infertility in both men and women.

2. Chasteberry: Chasteberry is a small, purple berry that has been used to treat infertility in women for many years. It contains compounds that can help to regulate hormones and improve ovulation.

3. Maca Root: Maca root is a plant that is native to the Andes Mountains in South America. It has been used to boost fertility in both men and women due to its high levels of nutrients and antioxidants.

4. Ginseng: Ginseng is an herb that has been used for centuries to treat a variety of health issues, including infertility. It can help to boost fertility by regulating hormones and improving the quality of sperm.

5. Saw Palmetto: Saw Palmetto is an herb that has been used for centuries to improve fertility in both men and women. It can help to increase libido, improve sperm production, and regulate hormones.

6. Ashwagandha: Ashwagandha is an Ayurvedic herb that has been used for centuries to treat infertility. It can help to regulate hormones, improve sperm count, and improve egg quality.

7. Dandelion Root: Dandelion root is an herb that is high in vitamins and minerals. It has been used to treat infertility due to its ability to improve liver function and regulate hormones.

8. Tribulus Terrestris: Tribulus Terrestris is an herb that has been used for centuries to improve fertility in both men and women. It can help to increase testosterone levels, improve sperm count, and boost libido.

9. Stinging Nettle: Stinging nettle is an herb that has been used for centuries to treat infertility. It can help to improve hormone balance and boost fertility by increasing sperm count and improving egg quality.

10. Fennel: Fennel is an herb that has been used for centuries to improve fertility in both men and women. It can help to increase libido, regulate hormones, and improve sperm quality.

CHAPTER 8

FERTILITY RECIPES

BREAKFAST

1. Omelet with Avocado, Tomato, and Cheese:

Ingredients:

- 2 eggs
- 2 tablespoons milk
- 1/4 teaspoon salt
- 1/4 teaspoon ground black pepper
- 2 tablespoons olive oil
- 1/2 avocado, sliced
- 1/4 cup cherry or grape tomatoes, cleaned and halved
- 1/4 cup shredded cheese

Instructions:

1. Combine the eggs, milk, salt, and pepper in a medium bowl.
2. In a medium nonstick skillet over medium heat, warm the olive oil.
3. Pour the egg mixture into the skillet and cook until the edges are set and the center is still slightly runny, about 4 minutes.
4. Add the avocado, tomatoes, and cheese to one half of the omelet.

5. Fold the other half of the omelet over the filling and cook until the cheese is melted and the eggs are cooked through, about 2 minutes.
6. Toast should be served alongside the omelet.

Prep Time: 10 minutes

2. French Toast with Nut Butter and Berries:

Ingredients:

- 2 slices whole-grain bread
- 2 eggs
- 2 tablespoons milk
- 1 tablespoon butter
- 2 tablespoons nut butter
- 1/2 cup fresh or frozen berries

Instructions:

1. Eggs and milk should be whisked together in a shallow bowl.
2. In a nonstick skillet over medium heat, melt the butter.
3. Bread slices are dipped in the egg mixture and both sides are coated. Place in the skillet and cook until golden brown, about 2 minutes per side.
4. Spread each slice with nut butter and top with the berries.
5. Drizzle some maple syrup over the French toast before serving.

Prep Time: 10 minutes

3. Scrambled Eggs with Spinach and Feta:

Ingredients:

- 2 eggs
- 2 tablespoons milk
- 1 tablespoon butter
- 1/2 cup spinach, chopped
- 2 tablespoons feta cheese, crumbled
- Salt and pepper, to taste

Instructions:

1. In a medium bowl, whisk together the eggs and milk.
2. Heat the butter in a non-stick skillet over medium heat.
3. Add the egg mixture to the skillet and cook, stirring often, until the eggs are almost set.
4. Add the spinach and feta cheese and cook until the eggs are cooked through.
5. Season with salt and pepper, to taste.
6. Serve the scrambled eggs with a side of toast.

Prep Time: 10 minutes

4. Yogurt Bowl with Granola and Honey:

Ingredients:

- 1 cup plain Greek yogurt
- 1/4 cup granola
- 2 tablespoons honey
- 1/4 cup fresh or frozen berries

Instructions:

1. In a bowl, combine the yogurt, granola, and honey.
2. Top with the berries.
3. Serve the yogurt bowl with a drizzle of extra honey, if desired.

Prep Time: 5 minutes

5. Breakfast Smoothie Bowl:

Ingredients:

- 1 frozen banana
- 1/2 cup frozen strawberries
- 1/4 cup almond milk
- 2 tablespoons chia seeds
- 2 tablespoons ground flaxseed
- 2 tablespoons almond butter
- 1/4 cup granola

Instructions:

1. Place the banana, strawberries, almond milk, chia seeds, and flaxseed in a blender and blend until smooth.
2. Pour the smoothie into a bowl and top with the almond butter and granola.
3. Serve the smoothie bowl with extra almond butter and granola, if desired.

Prep Time: 10 minutes

6. Overnight Oats with Berries:

Ingredients:

- 1/2 cup rolled oats
- 1/2 cup milk
- 2 tablespoons chia seeds
- 2 tablespoons honey
- 1/4 cup fresh or frozen berries

Instructions:

1. In a bowl, combine the oats, milk, chia seeds, and honey.
2. Cover and refrigerate overnight.
3. In the morning, top the oats with the berries.
4. Serve the overnight oats with a drizzle of honey, if desired.

Prep Time: 10 minutes

7. Breakfast Burrito with Eggs and Black Beans:

Ingredients:

- 2 eggs
- 2 tablespoons milk
- 1/4 teaspoon salt
- 1/4 teaspoon ground black pepper
- 2 tablespoons olive oil
- 1/2 cup cooked black beans
- 1/4 cup shredded cheese
- 2 tablespoons salsa
- 2 small tortillas

Instructions:

1. In a medium bowl, whisk together the eggs, milk, salt, and pepper.
2. Heat the olive oil in a medium non-stick skillet over medium heat.
3. Pour the egg mixture into the skillet and cook until the edges are set and the center is still slightly runny, about 4 minutes.
4. Divide the eggs, black beans, cheese, and salsa evenly between the tortillas.
5. Roll up the burritos and serve.

Prep Time: 10 minutes

8. Apple-Cinnamon Oatmeal:

Ingredients:

- 1/2 cup rolled oats
- 1 cup milk
- 1/2 apple, diced
- 1/2 teaspoon ground cinnamon
- 2 tablespoons honey

Instructions:

1. In a small saucepan, combine the oats and milk.
2. Bring to a boil over medium heat, stirring often.
3. Reduce heat to low and simmer, stirring often, until the oats are cooked through, about 5 minutes.
4. Stir in the apple, cinnamon, and honey and cook until the apple is tender, about 2 minutes.
5. Serve the oatmeal with a drizzle of honey, if desired.

Prep Time: 10 minutes

9. Breakfast Quesadilla with Eggs and Peppers:

Ingredients:

- 2 eggs
- 2 tablespoons milk
- 1/4 teaspoon salt
- 1/4 teaspoon ground black pepper
- 2 tablespoons olive oil
- 1/4 cup diced bell peppers
- 1/4 cup shredded cheese
- 2 small tortillas

Instructions:

1. In a medium bowl, whisk together the eggs, milk, salt, and pepper.
2. Heat the olive oil in a medium non-stick skillet over medium heat.
3. Pour the egg mixture into the skillet and cook until the edges are set and the center is still slightly runny, about 4 minutes.
4. Divide the eggs, bell peppers, and cheese evenly between the tortillas.
5. Fold the tortillas in half and cook until the cheese is melted and the eggs are cooked through, about 2 minutes per side.
6. Serve the quesadillas with a side of salsa.

Prep Time: 10 minutes

10. Egg Muffins with Spinach and Cheese:

Ingredients:

- 6 eggs
- 1/4 cup milk
- 1/4 teaspoon salt
- 1/4 teaspoon ground black pepper
- 2 tablespoons olive oil
- 1/2 cup spinach, chopped
- 1/4 cup shredded cheese

Instructions:

1. Preheat oven to 350°F. Grease a 12-cup muffin pan with cooking spray.
2. In a medium bowl, whisk together the eggs, milk, salt, and pepper.
3. Heat the olive oil in a medium non-stick skillet over medium heat.
4. Pour the egg mixture into the skillet and cook until the edges are set, about 2 minutes.
5. Divide the eggs, spinach, and cheese evenly among the muffin cups.
6. Bake until the eggs are cooked through, about 10 minutes.
7. Serve the egg muffins warm.

Prep Time: 10 minutes

LUNCH

1. Mediterranean Quinoa Bowl - Prep time: 15 minutes

Ingredients:

- 1 cup of cooked quinoa
- 1/2 cup of diced cherry tomatoes
- 1/4 cup of crumbled feta cheese
- 1/4 cup of diced cucumber
- 1/4 cup of diced red onion
- 1/4 cup of kalamata olives
- 1/4 cup of chopped fresh parsley
- 2 tablespoons of olive oil
- 1 tablespoon of lemon juice that has just been squeezed
- Salt and pepper to taste

Instructions:

1. Prepare the quinoa as directed on the package.
2. In a large bowl, combine the cooked quinoa, tomatoes, feta cheese, cucumber, red onion, olives, and parsley.
3. In a small bowl, whisk together the olive oil, lemon juice, salt, and pepper.
4. Pour the dressing over the quinoa mixture and stir until evenly combined.
5. Serve the quinoa bowl warm or cold.

2. Thai Peanut Noodle Bowl - Prep time: 15 minutes

Ingredients:

- 1 package of cooked soba noodles
- 1 cup of shredded cooked chicken
- 1/2 cup of chopped red bell pepper
- 1/2 cup of shredded carrots
- 1/4 cup of chopped scallions
- 2 tablespoons of peanut butter
- 2 tablespoons of soy sauce
- 1 tablespoon of rice vinegar
- 1 teaspoon of sesame oil
- 1 teaspoon of grated ginger

Instructions:

1. Prepare the soba noodles as directed on the packet.
2. In a large bowl, combine the cooked noodles, chicken, bell pepper, carrots, and scallions.
3. In a small bowl, whisk together the peanut butter, soy sauce, rice vinegar, sesame oil, and ginger.
4. Pour the dressing over the noodle mixture and stir until evenly combined.
5. Serve the noodle bowl warm or cold.

3. Egg and Avocado Toast: Prep time: 10 minutes

Ingredients:

- 2 slices of whole wheat bread
- 2 eggs

- 1 avocado
- 1 tablespoon of olive oil
- 1 tablespoon of lemon juice that has just been squeezed
- Salt and pepper to taste

Instructions:

1. Toast the slices of bread till golden brown.
2. Heat the olive oil in a skillet over medium heat.
3. Add salt and pepper to the skillet with the cracked eggs. Cook until the yolks are still runny but the whites are set.
4. In a small bowl, mash the avocado with the lemon juice.
5. Spread the avocado onto the toast slices.
6. Top the toast with the cooked eggs.
7. Serve the egg and avocado toast warm.

4. Lemon Garlic Shrimp: Prep time: 10 minutes

Ingredients:

- One pound of peeled and deveined shrimp
- 2 tablespoons of olive oil
- 2 cloves of garlic, minced
- 2 teaspoons of lemon juice that has just been squeezed
- 2 tablespoons of chopped fresh parsley
- Salt and pepper to taste

Instructions:

1. Place a large skillet over medium heat and add the olive oil.
2. Add the shrimp and garlic to the skillet and cook until the shrimp are pink and cooked through.

3. Remove the skillet from the heat and stir in the lemon juice, parsley, salt, and pepper.
4. Serve the shrimp warm.

5. Greek Salad Bowl - Prep time: 10 minutes

Ingredients:

- 1/2 cup of cooked quinoa
- 1/2 cup of diced cucumber
- 1/4 cup of diced red onion
- 1/4 cup of kalamata olives
- 1/4 cup of crumbled feta cheese
- 2 teaspoons of lemon juice that has just been squeezed
- 2 tablespoons of olive oil
- 1 tablespoon of chopped fresh oregano
- Salt and pepper to taste

Instructions:

1. In a large bowl, combine the quinoa, cucumber, red onion, olives, and feta cheese.
2. Combine the lemon juice, olive oil, oregano, salt, and pepper in a small bowl.
3. Pour the dressing over the quinoa mixture and stir until evenly combined.
4. Serve the Greek salad bowl warm or cold.

6. Grilled Vegetable Wrap: Prep time: 15 minutes

Ingredients:

- 2 whole wheat tortillas
- 1/2 cup of grilled vegetables (such as bell peppers, onions, and zucchini)
- 1/4 cup of crumbled feta cheese
- 2 tablespoons of olive oil
- 1 tablespoon of lemon juice that has just been squeezed
- Salt and pepper to taste

Instructions:

1. Turn on the medium heat and prepare a grill or grill pan.
2. Grill the vegetables until lightly charred and tender.
3. In a small bowl, whisk together the olive oil, lemon juice, salt, and pepper.
4. Spread the dressing onto the tortillas.
5. Top the tortillas with the grilled vegetables and feta cheese.
6. Roll up the tortillas and cut in half.
7. Serve the vegetable wraps warm.

7. Baked Sweet Potato - Prep time: 10 minutes

Ingredients:

- 1 large sweet potato
- 2 tablespoons of olive oil
- 1 tablespoon of lemon juice that has just been squeezed
- 1 teaspoon of chopped fresh rosemary

- Salt and pepper to taste

Instructions:

1. Set the oven's temperature to 400 degrees.
2. Use a fork to pierce the sweet potato all over.
3. Rub the sweet potato with the olive oil, lemon juice, rosemary, salt, and pepper.
4. Put a baking sheet with the sweet potato in it.
5. Bake for 40-45 minutes, or until the sweet potato is tender.
6. Serve the baked sweet potato warm.

8. Avocado Toast with Fried Egg - Prep time: 10 minutes

Ingredients:

- 2 slices of whole wheat bread
- 1 avocado
- 2 eggs
- 1 tablespoon of olive oil
- 1 tablespoon of freshly squeezed lemon juice
- Salt and pepper to taste

Instructions:

1. Toast the slices of bread till golden brown.
2. Heat the olive oil in a skillet over medium heat.
3. Add salt and pepper to the skillet with the cracked eggs. Cook until the yolks are still runny but the whites are set.
4. In a small bowl, mash the avocado with the lemon juice.
5. Spread the avocado onto the toast slices.
6. Top the toast with the fried eggs.

7. Serve the avocado toast with fried egg warm.

9. Chickpea Salad - Prep time: 10 minutes

Ingredients:
- 1 can of washed and drained chickpeas
- 1/2 cup of diced cucumber
- 1/4 cup of diced red onion
- 1/4 cup of chopped fresh parsley
- 2 tablespoons of olive oil
- 1 tablespoon of lemon juice that has just been squeezed
- Salt and pepper to taste

Instructions:
1. In a large bowl, combine the chickpeas, cucumber, red onion, and parsley.
2. Combine the olive oil, lemon juice, salt, and pepper in a small bowl.
3. Pour the dressing over the chickpea mixture and stir until evenly combined.
4. Serve the chickpea salad warm or cold.

10. Roasted Vegetable Bowl - Prep time: 20 minutes

Ingredients:
- 1 cup of chopped vegetables (such as bell peppers, onions, and zucchini)
- 2 tablespoons of olive oil

- 1 tablespoon of lemon juice that has just been squeezed
- 1 teaspoon of chopped fresh oregano
- Salt and pepper to taste

Instructions:

1. Set the oven's temperature to 400 degrees.
2. In a baking dish, combine the vegetables and olive oil.
3. Roast the vegetables in the oven for 15-20 minutes, or until tender.
4. In a small bowl, whisk together the lemon juice, oregano, salt, and pepper.
5. Pour the dressing over the roasted vegetables and stir until evenly combined.
6. Serve the roasted vegetable bowl warm.

DINNER

1. Pesto Chicken, Tomato, and Asparagus Skewers – Prep Time: 15 minutes

Ingredients:

- 2 large boneless, skinless chicken breasts, cut into cubes
- 1/2 cup prepared pesto
- 1/4 cup olive oil
- 2 cups cherry tomatoes
- 2 cups asparagus spears
- Salt and pepper to taste

Instructions:

- Preheat the oven to 375°F.
- In a large bowl, combine the chicken cubes, pesto, and olive oil. Mix to combine.
- Place the chicken cubes, tomatoes, and asparagus onto metal skewers. Sprinkle with salt and pepper.
- Place the skewers onto a baking sheet and bake for 15 minutes, or until the chicken is cooked through.

2. Feta and Spinach Stuffed Mushrooms – Prep Time: 15 minutes

Ingredients:

- 12 large white mushrooms
- 1 tablespoon olive oil
- 1/2 cup feta cheese, crumbled
- 1 cup baby spinach
- 1 tablespoon minced garlic
- Salt and pepper to taste

Instructions:

- Preheat the oven to 375°F.
- Cut the mushroom stems off and throw them away.
- In a medium bowl, combine the feta cheese, spinach, garlic, salt, and pepper. Mix until well combined.
- Stuff each mushroom cap with the feta and spinach mixture.
- Place the mushrooms onto a baking sheet and bake for 15 minutes, or until the mushrooms are tender.

3. Baked Salmon with Herbed Yogurt Sauce – Prep Time: 10 minutes

Ingredients:

- 2 6-ounce salmon fillets

- 2 tablespoons olive oil
- Salt and pepper to taste
- 1/2 cup plain Greek yogurt
- 1 teaspoon fresh dill
- 1 teaspoon fresh parsley
- 1 teaspoon fresh chives

Instructions:

- Preheat the oven to 375°F.
- Place the salmon fillets onto a baking sheet. Sprinkle the salmon with salt and pepper, drizzle with olive oil, and bake for 10 minutes, or until the fish is thoroughly cooked.
- In a small bowl, combine the yogurt, dill, parsley, and chives. Mix to combine.
- Serve the salmon with the herbed yogurt sauce.

4. Eggplant Parmesan – Prep Time: 15 minutes

Ingredients:

- 2 large eggplants, sliced
- 1/4 cup olive oil
- 2 cups marinara sauce
- 1 cup shredded mozzarella cheese

- 1/2 cup grated Parmesan cheese
- Salt and pepper to taste

Instructions:

- Preheat the oven to 375°F.
- Place the eggplant slices onto a baking sheet and drizzle with olive oil. Sprinkle with salt and pepper.
- Bake for 15 minutes, or until the eggplant is tender.
- Spread the marinara sauce onto the eggplant slices. Top with the mozzarella and Parmesan cheeses.
- Bake for an additional 10 minutes, or until the cheese is melted and bubbly.

5. Baked Cod with Lemon and Parsley – Prep Time: 15 minutes

Ingredients:

- 2 6-ounce cod fillets
- 2 tablespoons olive oil
- Juice of 1 lemon
- 2 tablespoons chopped fresh parsley
- Salt and pepper to taste

Instructions:

- Preheat the oven to 375°F.

- Place the cod fillets onto a baking sheet. Sprinkle with salt and pepper and drizzle with olive oil.
- Bake for 10 minutes, or until the cod is cooked through.
- Squeeze the lemon juice over the cod and sprinkle with parsley.
- Bake for an additional 5 minutes, or until the lemon juice is cooked into the cod.

6. Roasted Sweet Potato Salad – Prep Time: 20 minutes

Ingredients:

- Two big sweet potatoes, diced and peeled
- 2 tablespoons olive oil
- 1 red bell pepper, diced
- 1/2 red onion, diced
- 1/4 cup crumbled feta cheese
- 2 tablespoons chopped fresh parsley
- 2 tablespoons red wine vinegar
- Salt and pepper to taste

Instructions:

- Preheat the oven to 375°F.
- Place the sweet potatoes onto a baking sheet and drizzle with olive oil.

- Roast the sweet potatoes for 20 minutes, or until they are cooked through.
- In a large bowl, combine the roasted sweet potatoes, bell pepper, onion, feta cheese, and parsley.
- Sprinkle with salt and pepper and drizzle with red wine vinegar.
- Serve warm or chilled.

7. Zucchini Noodles with Tomato Alfredo Sauce – Prep Time: 10 minutes

Ingredients:

- 2 large zucchinis, spiralized
- 2 tablespoons olive oil
- 2 cloves garlic, minced
- 1/2 cup heavy cream
- 1 cup marinara sauce
- 1/2 cup grated Parmesan cheese
- Salt and pepper to taste

Instructions:

- In a sizable skillet set over medium heat, warm the olive oil.
- After adding it, sauté the garlic for one minute, or until fragrant.
- Add the heavy cream and marinara sauce and bring to a simmer.
- Add the Parmesan cheese after lowering the heat to a low setting. 5 minutes of simmering should be plenty to thicken the sauce.

- Add the zucchini noodles to the skillet and toss to coat in the sauce. Cook for 2 minutes, or until the noodles are tender.
- Serve after seasoning with salt and pepper.

8. Garlic Butter Shrimp – Prep Time: 10 minutes

Ingredients:

- 2 tablespoons butter
- 2 cloves garlic, minced
- 1/4 teaspoon red pepper flakes
- 1 pound shrimp, peeled and deveined
- 2 tablespoons fresh lemon juice
- Salt and pepper to taste

Instructions:

- In a large skillet over medium heat, melt the butter.
- Add the garlic and red pepper flakes and sauté, stirring occasionally, for 1 minute, or until fragrant.
- Add the shrimp and cook for 2 minutes, or until the shrimp is cooked through.
- Add the lemon juice and season with salt and pepper.
- Serve warm.

9. Baked Zucchini Fritters – Prep Time: 15 minutes

Ingredients:

- 2 large zucchini, grated

- 1/2 cup all-purpose flour
- 2 tablespoons grated Parmesan cheese
- 1 tablespoon minced garlic
- 1 egg, lightly beaten
- Salt and pepper to taste

Instructions:

- Preheat the oven to 375°F.
- In a large bowl, combine the grated zucchini, flour, Parmesan cheese, garlic, egg, salt, and pepper. Mix until well combined.
- Form the mixture into small patties and place onto a baking sheet.
- Bake for 15 minutes, or until the fritters are golden brown.

10. Baked Tofu with Sweet and Spicy Glaze – Prep Time: 10 minutes

Ingredients:

- 1 block extra-firm tofu, drained and cubed
- 2 tablespoons olive oil
- 2 tablespoons soy sauce
- 2 tablespoons honey
- 1 tablespoon rice vinegar
- 1 tablespoon sesame seeds
- 1 teaspoon sriracha
- Salt and pepper to taste

Instructions:

- Preheat the oven to 375°F.

- Place the tofu cubes onto a baking sheet and drizzle with olive oil.
- In a small bowl, combine the soy sauce, honey, rice vinegar, sesame seeds, and sriracha. Mix until well combined.
- Pour the glaze over the tofu and toss to coat. Sprinkle with salt and pepper.
- Bake for 10 minutes, or until the tofu is golden brown.

SNACK

1. Avocado and Egg Toast:

This simple snack is a great way to get a protein and healthy fat boost in a single bite.

Ingredients:

- 2 slices of whole grain bread
- 2 eggs
- 1 avocado, peeled and mashed
- 1/4 teaspoon of salt
- 2 tablespoons of olive oil

Preparation:

- Place a skillet with the olive oil over medium heat.
- Add the eggs and cook for about 3 minutes, flipping once, until the whites are cooked through.
- Meanwhile, toast the bread and spread the mashed avocado onto each slice.
- When the eggs are done, season with salt and place them on top of the avocado toast.

Prep Time: 10 minutes

2. Apple and Cheese Skewers:

These bite size snacks are a great way to get some calcium, protein, and fruit all in one.

Ingredients:

- 2 apples, cut into wedges
- Four ounces of cubed cheddar cheese
- 1 tablespoon of honey
- 2 tablespoons of olive oil
- 1/4 teaspoon of salt

Preparation:

- Place a skillet with the olive oil over medium heat.
- Place the apple wedges and cheese cubes onto skewers.
- Place the skewers in the skillet and cook for about 3 minutes, flipping once, until the cheese is melted and the apples are slightly softened.
- Drizzle with honey and season with salt.

Prep Time: 10 minutes

3. Greek Yogurt and Fruit Parfait:

This nutrient-packed snack is a great way to get a boost of calcium and vitamins.

Ingredients:

- 1 cup of plain Greek yogurt
- Chopped 1/2 cup of your preferred fruit
- 2 tablespoons of honey
- 2 tablespoons of chopped almonds

Preparation:

- Place the yogurt in a bowl.
- Layer the chopped fruit, honey, and almonds on top.

- Serve and enjoy!

Prep Time: 5 minutes

4. Trail Mix:

This snack is a great way to get a variety of nutrients and energy in a single scoop.

Ingredients:
- 1/2 cup of roasted almonds
- 1/2 cup of dried cranberries
- 1/4 cup of dark chocolate chips
- 1/4 cup of pumpkin seeds
- 2 tablespoons of flaxseeds

Preparation:
- In a bowl, combine all the ingredients.
- Store in an airtight container.
- Enjoy whenever you need an energy boost!

Prep Time: 5 minutes

5. Hummus and Veggies:

This savory snack is a great way to get some fiber, healthy fats, and vitamins in one bite.

Ingredients:
- 1/2 cup of hummus
- Chopped 1/2 cup of your preferred vegetables
- 2 tablespoons of olive oil

- 1/4 teaspoon of salt

Preparation:

- Spread the hummus onto a plate.
- Top with the chopped vegetables.
- Drizzle with olive oil and season with salt.
- Enjoy!

Prep Time: 5 minutes

6. Peanut Butter and Banana Toast:

This protein-packed snack is a great way to get a quick energy boost.

Ingredients:

- 2 slices of whole grain bread
- 2 tablespoons of peanut butter
- 1 banana, sliced
- 2 tablespoons of honey

Preparation:

- Toast the bread and spread the peanut butter onto each slice.
- Top with the banana slices and drizzle with honey.
- Serve and enjoy!

Prep Time: 5 minutes

7. Quinoa and Veggies:

This nutrient-packed snack is a great way to get some fiber and vitamins all in one bite.

Ingredients:

- 1/2 cup of cooked quinoa
- Chopped 1/2 cup of your preferred vegetables
- 2 tablespoons of olive oil
- 1/4 teaspoon of salt

Preparation:

- Place a skillet with the olive oil over medium heat.
- Add the quinoa and vegetables and cook for about 5 minutes, stirring occasionally, until the vegetables are tender.
- Season with salt and serve.

Prep Time: 10 minutes

8. Dark Chocolate and Almond Butter Bites:

These bite-size snacks are a great way to get a healthy dose of antioxidants and healthy fats.

Ingredients:

- 2 ounces of dark chocolate, chopped
- 1/4 cup of almond butter
- 1/4 cup of chopped almonds

Preparation:

- Line a baking sheet with parchment paper.
- Place the chopped chocolate and almond butter in a microwave-safe bowl and heat for about 30 seconds, stirring every 10 seconds, until melted.
- Stir in the almonds and spoon the mixture onto the baking sheet.
- Place the baking sheet in the refrigerator for about 10 minutes, until the bites are set.
- Serve and enjoy!

Prep Time: 15 minutes

9. Smoothie:

This nutrient-packed smoothie is a great way to get a quick energy boost.

Ingredients:

- 1 banana
- 1/2 cup of frozen berries
- 1/2 cup of plain Greek yogurt
- 1/4 cup of milk
- 1 tablespoon of honey

Preparation:

- Blend each item in the blender until it is smooth.
- Serve and enjoy!

Prep Time: 5 minutes

10. Avocado Toast with Egg:

This savory snack is a great way to get a protein and healthy fat boost in a single bite.

Ingredients:

- 2 slices of whole grain bread
- 2 eggs
- 1 avocado, peeled and mashed
- 2 tablespoons of olive oil
- 1/4 teaspoon of salt

Preparation:

- Place a skillet with the olive oil over medium heat.
- Add the eggs and cook for about 3 minutes, flipping once, until the whites are cooked through.
- Meanwhile, toast the bread and spread the mashed avocado onto each slice.
- When the eggs are done, season with salt and place them on top of the avocado toast.

Prep Time: 10 minutes

DESSERTS

1. Carrot Cake Cupcakes with Cream Cheese Frosting:

Introduction: Carrot cake cupcakes with creamy cream cheese frosting are the perfect way to celebrate a special occasion. These delicious treats are easy to make and sure to be a hit.

Ingredients:

2 cups all-purpose flour, 2 teaspoons baking powder, 2 teaspoons ground cinnamon, 1 teaspoon ground ginger, 1/4 teaspoon ground nutmeg, 1/2 teaspoon baking soda, 1/2 teaspoon salt, 1 1/2 cups granulated sugar, 1/2 cup vegetable oil, 2 large eggs, 1 teaspoon pure vanilla extract, 1 1/2 cups grated carrots, 1/2 cup chopped walnuts, 8 ounces cream cheese, 1/2 cup unsalted butter, 2 cups confectioners' sugar.

Preparation Method:

Preheat oven to 350 degrees F and line a 12-cup muffin pan with baking cups. Mix the flour with the baking powder, salt, nutmeg, ginger, cinnamon, and baking soda in a medium bowl. In a separate bowl, beat together the sugar, oil, eggs and vanilla until smooth. Stir in the carrots and walnuts. Beat in the flour mixture until barely incorporated after adding it. Incorporate the batter into the muffin tins as desired. A toothpick put into the center of a cupcake should come out clean after 20 minutes of baking. Let cool completely.

For the frosting, beat together the cream cheese and butter in a medium bowl until light and fluffy. Beat while gradually adding confectioners' sugar until smooth. After the cupcakes have cooled, top them with icing.

Prep Time: 30 minutes

2. Chocolate Chip Cookie Cake:

Introduction: This decadent and indulgent chocolate chip cookie cake is the perfect way to celebrate a special occasion. The combination of rich chocolate chips and creamy frosting is sure to satisfy any sweet tooth!

Ingredients:

3/4 cup butter, softened, 1 1/4 cups packed brown sugar, 2 eggs, 1 teaspoon vanilla extract, 2 1/4 cups all-purpose flour, 1 teaspoon baking soda, 1/2 teaspoon salt, 2 cups semisweet chocolate chips, 2 cups whipping cream, 1/2 cup confectioners' sugar.

Preparation Method:

Preheat oven to 375 degrees F and grease a 9-inch round cake pan. In a medium bowl, beat together the butter and brown sugar until light and fluffy. Mix the eggs and vanilla thoroughly before adding them. Mix the flour, baking soda, and salt in a separate bowl. Gradually add the flour mixture to the butter mixture and beat until just combined. Stir in the chocolate chips. On the prepared cake pan, spread the batter. A toothpick put into the center of the cake should come out clean after 20 minutes of baking. Let cool completely.

For the frosting, beat the cream and confectioners' sugar in a medium bowl until thick and creamy. Spread the frosting over the cooled cake.

Prep Time: 45 minutes

3. Apple Pie Bars:

Introduction: These delicious and easy-to-make apple pie bars are the perfect way to satisfy your sweet tooth. The combination of warm cinnamon, juicy apples and a sweet crumb topping is sure to please!

Ingredients:

2 cups all-purpose flour, 1/2 cup granulated sugar, 1/2 cup packed brown sugar, 1 teaspoon ground cinnamon, 1/2 teaspoon ground nutmeg, 1/2 teaspoon baking soda, 1/2 teaspoon salt, 1 cup cold butter, cut into small cubes, 4 cups peeled and thinly sliced apples, 1/2 cup water, 2 tablespoons cornstarch, 1/3 cup packed brown sugar, 1/2 teaspoon ground cinnamon, 1/4 teaspoon ground nutmeg.

Preparation Method:

Grease a 9 x 13-inch baking dish and preheat the oven to 350 degrees F. In a medium bowl, whisk together the flour, granulated sugar, brown sugar, cinnamon, nutmeg, baking soda and salt. Butter should be incorporated into the mixture until it resembles coarse crumbs. Press half of the mixture into the prepared pan.

In a medium saucepan, combine the apples, water, cornstarch, brown sugar, cinnamon, and nutmeg. Bring to a boil, stirring occasionally. Reduce heat and simmer until the apples are tender, about 5 minutes. Pour the apples over the crust. Over the apples, scatter the remaining crumbs mixture. Bake for thirty minutes, or until golden brown on top. Let bars cool completely before slicing.

Prep Time: 45 minutes

4. Blueberry Cheesecake Bars:

Introduction: These creamy and delicious blueberry cheesecake bars are the perfect way to satisfy your sweet tooth. The combination of creamy cheesecake and sweet blueberries is sure to be a hit!

Ingredients:

2 cups graham cracker crumbs, 1/2 cup melted butter, 2 (8-ounce) packages cream cheese, softened, 1/2 cup granulated sugar, 2 large eggs, 2 teaspoons vanilla extract, 1/2 teaspoon salt, 1 cup sour cream, 2 cups fresh or frozen blueberries, 2 tablespoons cornstarch.

Preparation Method:

Grease a 9x13-inch baking dish and preheat the oven to 350 degrees Fahrenheit. In a medium bowl, combine the graham cracker crumbs and melted butter. Put some pressure on the prepared pan's bottom. Cream cheese and sugar should be combined in a different bowl and beaten until frothy. One at a time, beat in the eggs, then add the salt and vanilla. On the graham cracker crust, spread the cream cheese mixture.

In a medium saucepan, combine the sour cream, blueberries, and cornstarch. Boil the mixture for about 5 minutes, or until it boils and thickens, over medium heat. Spread the blueberry mixture over the cream cheese layer. Bake for thirty minutes, or until golden brown on top. Let bars cool completely before slicing.

Prep Time: 45 minutes

5. Strawberry Shortcake Trifle:

Introduction: This delicious strawberry shortcake trifle is the perfect way to celebrate a special occasion. The combination of sweet strawberries, fluffy cake and creamy filling is sure to please!

Ingredients:

1 (12-ounce) package pound cake, cubed, 2 tablespoons orange juice, 1 cup milk, 1 (3.4-ounce) package instant vanilla pudding mix, 1 (8-ounce) package cream cheese, softened, 1/2 cup granulated sugar, 1 teaspoon vanilla extract, 2 cups heavy cream, 1/4 cup confectioners' sugar, 2 cups sliced fresh strawberries.

Preparation Method:

In a medium bowl, combine the cubed pound cake and orange juice. Divide the cake between 4 (1-quart) trifle dishes. In a separate bowl, whisk together the milk and pudding mix until thickened. In another bowl, beat together the cream cheese and granulated sugar until light and fluffy. Beat in the vanilla.

In a medium bowl, beat together the cream and confectioners' sugar until stiff peaks form. Let bars cool completely before slicing. Spoon the cream cheese mixture over the cake. Top with the pudding mixture, then the strawberries. Cream cheese and whipped cream should be combined.

Prep Time: 1 hour 15 minutes

6. Banana Pudding Parfaits:

Introduction: These delicious and easy-to-make banana pudding parfaits are the perfect way to end a meal. The combination of creamy pudding, sweet bananas and crunchy cookies is sure to please!

Ingredients:

1 (3.4-ounce) package instant vanilla pudding mix, 2 cups milk, 1 (8-ounce) package cream cheese, softened, 1/2 cup granulated sugar, 1 teaspoon vanilla extract, 2 cups heavy cream, 1/4 cup confectioners' sugar, 4 ripe bananas, sliced, 1 (12-ounce) package vanilla wafers, crushed.

Preparation Method:

In a medium bowl, whisk together the pudding mix and milk until thickened. In another bowl, beat together the cream cheese and granulated sugar until light and fluffy. Beat in the vanilla.

In a medium bowl, beat together the cream and confectioners' sugar until stiff peaks form. Cream cheese and whipped cream should be combined.

To assemble the parfaits, layer the banana slices, cream cheese mixture, pudding and crushed vanilla wafers in 8 (8-ounce) parfait glasses. Before serving, place in the fridge for at least one hour.

Prep Time: 1 hour 15 minutes

7. Lemon Bars:

Introduction: These delicious and easy-to-make lemon bars are the perfect way to indulge your sweet tooth. The combination of tart lemon and sweet shortbread crust is sure to please!

Ingredients:

1 1/2 cups all-purpose flour, 1/2 cup confectioners' sugar, 1/2 cup cold butter, cut into small cubes, 1/4 teaspoon salt, 4 large eggs, 1 1/2 cups granulated sugar, 1/4 cup all-purpose flour, 1/2 cup fresh lemon juice, 1 teaspoon grated lemon zest, 1/4 teaspoon baking powder, 1/4 teaspoon baking soda.

Preparation Method:

Grease a 9x13-inch baking dish and preheat the oven to 350 degrees Fahrenheit. In a medium bowl, whisk together the flour, confectioners' sugar, butter and salt until the mixture resembles coarse crumbs. Put some pressure on the prepared pan's bottom. Bake for 15 minutes, or until lightly browned.

In a separate bowl, whisk together the eggs, granulated sugar, flour, lemon juice, lemon zest, baking powder and baking soda until smooth. Pour over the prepared crust. 25 minutes of baking is required to lightly brown the top. Let bars cool completely before slicing.

Prep Time: 40 minutes

8. Raspberry Truffles:

Introduction: These delicious and easy-to-make raspberry truffles are the perfect way to satisfy your sweet tooth. The combination of creamy chocolate, tart raspberry and crunchy nuts is sure to please!

Ingredients:

1 (12-ounce) package semi-sweet chocolate chips, 1 (14-ounce) can sweetened condensed milk, 1 teaspoon vanilla extract, 1/2 teaspoon almond extract, 3 tablespoons raspberry preserves, 1/2 cup finely chopped almonds.

Preparation Method:

In a medium saucepan, melt the chocolate chips over low heat, stirring constantly. Slowly stir in the condensed milk and stir until smooth. Remove from heat and stir in the vanilla and almond extract.

Line a baking sheet with waxed paper. Drop the chocolate mixture by teaspoonfuls onto the waxed paper. Make an indentation in each truffle and fill with a teaspoon of raspberry preserves. Sprinkle with chopped almonds. Place in the fridge for one hour, or until firm.

Prep Time: 1 hour 15 minutes

9. Chocolate Mousse Cake:

Introduction: This decadent and delicious chocolate mousse cake is the perfect way to celebrate a special occasion. The combination of rich chocolate mousse and a light and fluffy cake is sure to please!

Ingredients:

1 (18.25-ounce) package devil's food cake mix, 1/2 cup vegetable oil, 2 large eggs, 2 cups cold water, 1 (3.9-ounce) package instant chocolate pudding mix, 2 cups cold milk, 1 (8-ounce) package cream cheese, softened, 1/2 cup granulated sugar, 2 teaspoons vanilla extract, 1 cup heavy cream, 1/4 cup confectioners' sugar.

Preparation Method:

Preheat oven to 350 degrees F and grease a 9-inch springform pan. In a medium bowl, whisk together the cake mix, oil, eggs and water until smooth. Pour into the prepared pan and bake for 25 minutes, or until a toothpick inserted into the center of the cake comes out clean. Let cool completely.

In a separate bowl, whisk together the pudding mix and milk until thickened. In another bowl, beat together the cream cheese and granulated sugar until light and fluffy. Beat in the vanilla.

In a medium bowl, beat together the cream and confectioners' sugar until stiff peaks form. Cream cheese and whipped cream should be combined. Spread the cream cheese mixture over the cooled cake. Cover the cream cheese layer with the pudding mixture. Before serving, place in the fridge for at least one hour.

Prep Time: 1 hour 15 minutes

10. Coconut Cream Pie:
Introduction: This delicious and easy-to-make coconut cream pie is the perfect way to end a meal. The combination of creamy coconut and sweet graham cracker crust is sure to please!

Ingredients:

1 cup sweetened shredded coconut, 1 (9-inch) prepared graham cracker crust, 1 (14-ounce) can sweetened condensed milk, 1/2 cup heavy cream, 2 large eggs, 1 teaspoon vanilla extract, 1/4 teaspoon ground nutmeg, 1/4 teaspoon ground cinnamon.

Preparation Method:

Preheat oven to 350 degrees F and spread the coconut evenly over a baking sheet. Bake for about 10 minutes, or until lightly toasted. Set aside.

In a medium bowl, whisk together the condensed milk, cream, eggs, vanilla, nutmeg and cinnamon until well combined. Stir in the toasted coconut. Pour the mixture into the prepared graham cracker crust. Bake for 25 minutes, or until set. Let cool completely before serving.

Prep Time: 45 minutes

SMOOTHIES

1. Berry Pomegranate Smoothie

Introduction: This fertility smoothie is packed with antioxidants and vitamins which can help boost fertility.

Ingredients: ¾ cup pomegranate juice, ½ cup frozen blueberries, ½ cup frozen raspberries, ½ cup plain yogurt, 1 tablespoon honey

Preparation: Blend each ingredient in a blender together until completely smooth.

Prep time: 5 minutes

2. Spinach Mango Smoothie

Introduction: This smoothie is a great source of folate, which is important for fertility.

Ingredients: ½ cup frozen mango chunks, ½ cup baby spinach, ½ cup plain yogurt, ½ cup almond milk, 1 tablespoon honey

Preparation: Blend each ingredient in a blender together until completely smooth.

Prep time: 5 minutes

3. Avocado Banana Smoothie

Introduction: This smoothie is rich in healthy fats and potassium, both of which help with fertility.

Ingredients: ½ ripe avocado, 1 banana, ½ cup almond milk, 1 tablespoon honey, ½ teaspoon vanilla extract

Preparation: Blend each ingredient in a blender together until completely smooth.

Prep time: 5 minutes

4. Chocolate Oats Smoothie

Introduction: This smoothie is a great source of iron which can help with fertility.

Ingredients: 1 cup almond milk, ½ cup rolled oats, 1 tablespoon cocoa powder, 1 tablespoon honey, ½ teaspoon vanilla extract

Preparation: Blend each ingredient in a blender together until completely smooth.

Prep time: 5 minutes

5. Orange Carrot Smoothie

Introduction: This smoothie is packed with beta-carotene and vitamin C, both of which can help with fertility.

Ingredients: 1 cup orange juice, ½ cup frozen carrots, ½ cup plain yogurt, 1 tablespoon honey

Preparation: Blend each ingredient in a blender together until completely smooth.

Prep time: 5 minutes

6. Peach Coconut Smoothie

Introduction: This smoothie is a great source of zinc, which is important for fertility.

Ingredients: ½ cup frozen peaches, ½ cup coconut milk, ½ cup plain yogurt, 1 tablespoon honey

Preparation: Blend each ingredient in a blender together until completely smooth.

Prep time: 5 minutes

7. Green Tea Smoothie

Introduction: This smoothie is rich in antioxidants and can help boost fertility.

Ingredients: ½ cup green tea, ½ cup frozen mango chunks, ½ cup plain yogurt, 1 tablespoon honey

Preparation: Blend each ingredient in a blender together until completely smooth.

Prep time: 5 minutes

8. Pineapple Coconut Smoothie

Introduction: This smoothie is a great source of vitamin C, which is important for fertility.

Ingredients: ½ cup frozen pineapple chunks, ½ cup coconut milk, ½ cup plain yogurt, 1 tablespoon honey

Preparation: Blend each ingredient in a blender together until completely smooth.

Prep time: 5 minutes

9. Apple Cinnamon Smoothie

Introduction: This smoothie is a great source of iron and can help with fertility.

Ingredients: 1 cup apple juice, ½ teaspoon ground cinnamon, ½ cup plain yogurt, 1 tablespoon honey

Preparation: Blend each ingredient in a blender together until completely smooth.

Prep time: 5 minutes

10. Banana Oat Smoothie

Introduction: This smoothie is packed with healthy fats and fiber, both of which can help with fertility.

Ingredients: 1 banana, ½ cup almond milk, ½ cup rolled oats, 1 tablespoon honey

Preparation: Blend each ingredient in a blender together until completely smooth.

Prep time: 5 minutes

CONCLUSION

Congratulations on completing your fertility diet cookbook!

In this cookbook, you've explored the many ways that a diet can help reduce inflammation, balance hormones and boost conception. You've learnt about the importance of incorporating anti-inflammatory foods, hormone-balancing foods, and fertility-boosting foods into your diet. Not only have you discovered some delicious recipes for breakfast, lunch, dinner and snacks, but you've also learnt about how to make the most of your diet to achieve your fertility goals.

We hope that this cookbook has been a useful resource for you as you embark on your fertility journey. With the right nutrition and lifestyle, you can create the best environment for conception to take place. Eating a nutrient-dense, anti-inflammatory diet, getting adequate sleep, reducing stress, and engaging in regular exercise can help you create a balanced, healthy lifestyle.

Remember to listen to your body and take the time to nourish yourself. Eating a fertility-friendly diet is just one part of the equation when it comes to fertility. Take time to nurture yourself with self-care practices, such as yoga, meditation, massage or relaxation techniques.

Most importantly, don't forget to enjoy the journey. Eating well and nourishing your body can be a fun and delicious experience. Have a little fun in the kitchen and get creative with the recipes in this cookbook. You're sure to enjoy the rewards of your efforts.

We wish you the absolute best of success as you pursue fertility. May you discover the joy and peace you seek.

Made in the USA
Las Vegas, NV
16 January 2025